Series editor
Daniel Horton-Szar
BSc (Hons)
United Medical and Dental
Schools of Guy's and
St Thomas's Hospitals
(UMDS),
London

Faculty advisor

(...omy)

Biomedical Science,
University of Sheffield

Musculoskeletal System

Sona V Biswas
BSc (Hons)
United Medical and
Dental Schools of Guy's
and St Thomas's
Hospitals (UMDS),
London

Rehana K Iqbal
BSc (Hons)
United Medical and
Dental Schools of Guy's
and St Thomas's
Hospitals (UMDS),
London

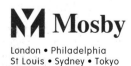

M Mosby

London • Philadelphia
St Louis • Sydney • Tokyo

Editor	**Louise Crowe**
Development Editor	**Filipa Maia**
Project Manager	**Louise Wilson**
Designer	**Greg Smith**
Layout	**Rob Curran**
Illustration Management	**Danny Pyne**
Illustrators	**Robin Dean**
	Deborah Gyan
	Danny Pyne
	Mike Saiz
	Marion Tasker
	Jeremy Theobold
	Amanda Williams
Cover Design	**Greg Smith**
Production	**Gudrun Hughes**
Index	**Janine Ross**

ISBN 0 7234 3127 2

Copyright © Mosby International Ltd, 1998.

Published by Mosby, an imprint of Mosby International Ltd, Lynton House, 7–12 Tavistock Square, London WC1H 9LB, UK.

Printed in Barcelona, Spain, by Grafos S.A. Arte sobre papel, 1998.
Text set in Crash Course—VAG Light; captions in Crash Course—VAG Thin.

Cataloguing in Publication Data
Catalogue records for this book are available from the British Library and the US Library of Congress.

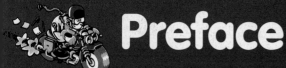

Preface

Crash Course Musculokeletal System aims to present a comprehensive overview of the musculoskeletal system in a clear and concise manner for medical students.

The preclinical aspects of anatomy, physiology, pharmacology, and pathology are integrated into a single system format in line with the new systems-based curricula that many medical schools teach. Clinical applications of the basic sciences relevant to the musculoskeletal system include the skills of history taking and examination, as well as some orthopaedics and rheumatology, covering common presenting complaints encountered by medical students in their clinical years.

The text has been compiled from our perspective as medical students. We hope you find it useful.

Good luck in your imminent exams.

Sona V Biswas
Rehana K Iqbal

This book on the musculoskeletal system, aimed at students in the preclinical years of their medical course, allows them to learn and revise the subject. *Crash Course Musculoskeletal System* provides a detailed yet concise guide through the structural organization, physiology, and pathology of the system, giving the reader sufficient information for a thorough understanding. The text is clearly presented mostly in bulleted form for easy comprehension and is supplemented with a number of informative illustrations.

Many medical schools now have fully integrated medical courses, but there are few textbooks to complement these recent changes in curricula. One of the difficulties experienced by today's medical students is the problem of finding relevant information from traditional textbooks which tend to include vast detail. Hence, there is a need for student-friendly books which cover pertinent topics whilst avoiding superfluous descriptions. *Crash Course Musculoskeletal System* is written by two medical students for their peers and more than meets these needs. It will enable the reader to master the basic science related to the musculoskeletal system and appreciate its relevance to medical practice.

Sam Jacob
Faculty Advisor

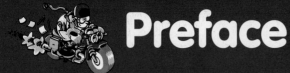 Preface

OK, no-one ever said medicine was going to be easy, but the thing is, there are very few parts of this enormous subject that are actually difficult to understand. The problem for most of us is the sheer volume of information that must be absorbed before each round of exams. It's not fun when time is getting short and you realize that: a) you really should have done a bit more work by now; and b) there are large gaps in your lecture notes that you meant to copy up but never quite got round to.

This series has been designed and written by senior medical students and doctors with recent experience of basic medical science exams. We've brought together all the information you need into compact, manageable volumes that integrate basic science with clinical skills. There is a consistent structure and layout across the series, and every title is checked for accuracy by senior faculty members from medical schools across the UK.

I hope this book makes things a little easier!

Danny Horton-Szar
Series Editor (Basic Medical Sciences)

Acknowledgements

SVB would like to thank D for telling her so, C for keeping her fed and watered, and M for helpful suggestions.

RKI would like to thank Rukhsana, Jared, Tara, Usma and Mehvish for all their help and support.

Both authors thank the team at Mosby, without whom this book would have been impossible.

Figure Credits

Figures 2.8b, 2.9, 2.10, 2.22, 3.6, 3.9a–c and 4.3 taken from *Human Histology 2e*, by A. Stevens and J. Lowe. Mosby, 1997. Figure 2.8b courtesy of Trevor Gray.

Figures 2.33, 2.39 and 3.17 taken from *McMinn's Functional and Clinical Anatomy*, by R.M.H. McMinn, P. Gaddum-Rosse, R.T. Hutchings and B.M. Logan. TMIP, 1995.

Figures 3.1, 7.6 and 7.9 taken from *Human Anatomy, Color Atlas and Text 3e* by J.A. Gosling, P.F. Harris, J.R. Humpherson, I. Whitmore and P.L.T. Wilan. TMIP, 1996.

Figures 3.13, 9.5, 10.1 and 10.2 from *Pathology* by A. Stevens and J. Lowe. Mosby, 1991.

Figure 3.3 from *Atlas of Orthopaedic Pathology* by P.G. Bullough, V.J. Vigorita and W.F. Enneking. Gower Medical Publishing, 1984.

Figures 1.3, 3.5, 3.11, 9.3, 9.6a and 10.9–10.11 from *Orthopaedic Pathology 3e* by P.G. Bullough and V.J. Vigorita. TMIP, 1997.

Figures 10.7, 10.8, 10.14, 10.15a, 10.20 and 10.23 taken from *Clinical Examination 2e* by O. Epstein, G.D. Perkin, D.P. de Bono and J. Cookson. Mosby 1997.

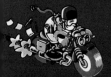

Contents

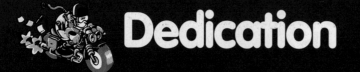

Dedication

To my family, **SVB**

To Mohammed Iqbal and Razub Akhtar, **RKI**

STRUCTURE AND FUNCTION OF THE MUSCULOSKELETAL SYSTEM

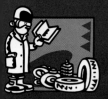

1. Musculoskeletal System — an Overview

Introduction
The musculoskeletal system comprises muscles, bones, and joints. It makes up most of the body's mass and performs several essential functions, including:
- The maintenance of body shape.
- The support and protection of soft tissue structures.
- Movement.
- Breathing.
- The storage of calcium and phosphate in bone.

Connective tissue
Most of the musculoskeletal system is made up of connective tissue such as bone and cartilage. Connective tissue comprises specialized cells embedded in an extracellular matrix of collagen, elastin, and structural proteoglycans. In bone, this matrix is mineralized and rigid.

Muscle
There are three types of muscle: skeletal, cardiac and smooth muscle.

Skeletal muscle
Skeletal muscle, which is striated muscle controlled by the nervous system. Most muscle in the body is of this type.

Cardiac muscle
Cardiac muscle, which is striated muscle of the heart.

Smooth muscle
Smooth muscle, which is non-striated muscle controlled by a variety of chemical mediators. Smooth muscle is important in the function of most tissues, for example, blood vessels, the gastrointestinal and reproductive tracts.

Energy stored as ATP is converted by muscle tissue into mechanical energy. This produces movement or tension.

The contraction of muscle requires stimulation. The type of stimulation varies: for example, skeletal muscle is activated by motor neurons, cardiac muscle initiates its own contractions, and smooth muscle is activated by a variety of chemical mediators. Stimulation of muscle causes actin and myosin, protein filaments within its cells, to interact, producing a contractile force.

The skeleton
The skeleton consists of bone, cartilage, and fibrous ligaments (p. 49). A joint is the site at which bones are attached to each other. A joint can be rigid or flexible depending on how the bones meet .

Bone
Bone is rigid and forms most of the skeleton. It provides a supportive framework for the musculoskeletal system, and sites for muscle attachment, the mechanical basis for locomotion. Other functions of bone include mineral storage in its matrix and formation of blood cells (haemopoiesis) within the marrow.

Cartilage
Cartilage is a resilient tissue that provides semi-rigid support in some parts of the skeleton. Cartilage is also a component of some types of joint. Most bone is formed within a cartilaginous template during development.

Ligaments, tendons, and aponeuroses
Ligaments, tendons, and aponeuroses are fibrous tissues that connect the various components of the musculoskeletal system.

Ligaments are flexible bands that connect bones or cartilage together, strengthening and stabilizing joints.

Tendons are connections between muscle and bone.

An aponeurosis may be considered as a broad, sheet-like tendon.

Joints
Joints are composite structures between bones. They may also include cartilage and fibrous connective tissue. There are several types of joint (p. 66). The strength of a joint and the range of movement it allows depend upon its position and function.

Control of the musculoskeletal system

The musculoskeletal system is controlled by the nervous system to produce coordinated movements and locomotion. There are a number of elements to this control. These include:

- Efferent motor neurons, which activate groups of muscle fibres to produce contraction.
- Afferent feedback from stretch receptors in muscles and tendons, and sensory nerve endings in joints and skin allowing coordination of movement.
- Neural pathways within the spinal cord, which coordinate the action of related muscle groups (agonist–antagonist pairs, for example) and also initiate repetitive actions, such as walking ('central pattern generator').

For further information about central control of movement and locomotion, refer to *Crash Course: Nervous System and Special Senses*.

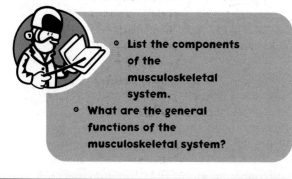

- List the components of the musculoskeletal system.
- What are the general functions of the musculoskeletal system?

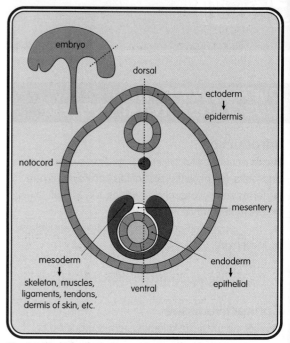

Fig. 1.1 The three primitive embryonic layers and their derivative structures.

- Mediating the exchange of nutrients and metabolic products between tissues and the circulatory system.
- Mechanical support, both physical as well as allowing for muscle attachment.
- Packaging, as connective tissue encloses and lies between other specialized tissues.
- A metabolic role, allowing fat storage in adipose tissue.
- Insulation.
- Defence and repair; some cells are involved in the immune response.

Components

The three main components of connective tissue are cells, fibres, and ground substance.

Cells

Connective tissue comprises several cell types. These cells each perform a certain function (Fig. 1.2).

Fibres

Collagen

Collagen is the main fibre found in the extracellular matrix of connective tissue. Collagen is produced from

CONNECTIVE TISSUE

Definition

Connective tissue is a basic type of tissue. It comprises cells embedded in an extracellular matrix of ground substance and fibres. Connective tissue is characterized by a high matrix:cell ratio.

Origins

Connective tissue is derived from the embryonic mesoderm and neural crest. These differentiate into the embryonic connective tissue or mesenchyme (Fig. 1.1).

Functions

Connective tissue performs several functions. These include:

tropocollagen, a substance synthesized by the endoplasmic reticulum of matrix-secreting cells. Tropocollagen becomes modified to collagen when it is released into the extracellular matrix.

Collagen comprises three helical polypeptide chains (Fig. 1.3). Differences in these chains result in at least 15 types of collagen molecules, each with a particular function (Fig. 1.4).

Elastin

Elastin is a component of elastic fibres. Elastic fibres are found in the skin, lung, and blood vessels. They are thinner than collagen and are arranged in random sheets.

Elastin is produced from proelastin, a substance synthesized by matrix-secreting cells. Proelastin becomes modified to elastin by the cell's Golgi apparatus, when it is released into the extracellular matrix.

Structural proteoglycans

Structural proteoglycans provide a ground substance surrounding the cells and fibres of connective tissue. They comprise protein chains bound to branched polysaccharides and form fibres such as fibronectin and laminin. Some structural proteoglycans are found on the surface of cells, where their functions include cell–cell recognition, adhesion, and migration.

Fig. 1.5 provides a classification of connective tissue.

Connective tissue cell types and functions		
	Cell type	**Functions**
fixed cells	fibroblasts, chondroblasts, osteoblasts, osteoclasts	synthesis and maintenance of matrix
	adipocytes	fat metabolism
	mast cells	release of histamine
	mesenchymal cells	mature cell precursors
transient cells	white blood cells	immune response
	melanocytes	pigmentation

Fig. 1.2 Connective tissue cell types and their functions.

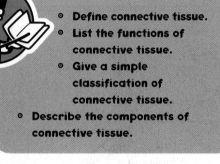

- Define connective tissue.
- List the functions of connective tissue.
- Give a simple classification of connective tissue.
- Describe the components of connective tissue.

Fig. 1.3 Microstructure of the collagen fibril. (A) Microfibril; (B) packing of molecules; (C) collagen molecule; and (D) triple helix of polypeptide (α) chains.

A fibril   microfibrils

B molecule packing

lacuna region   overlapping region

C

D

triple helical collagen molecule

280 nm

Functions of collagen types		
Type	Location	Function
I	skin, tendon, ligaments, bone, fascia and organ capsules (accounts for 90% of body collagen)	provides variable mechanical support (loose or dense)
II	hyaline and elastic cartilage, notochord, and intervertebral discs	provides shape and resistance to pressure
III	connective tissue of organs (liver, lymphoid organs, etc.), blood vessels, and fetal skin	forms reticular networks
IV	basement membrane of epithelial and endothelial cells	provides support and a filtration barrier
V	basement membrane of smooth and skeletal muscle cells	provides support (other functions poorly understood)

Fig. 1.4 Functions of the different types of collagen.

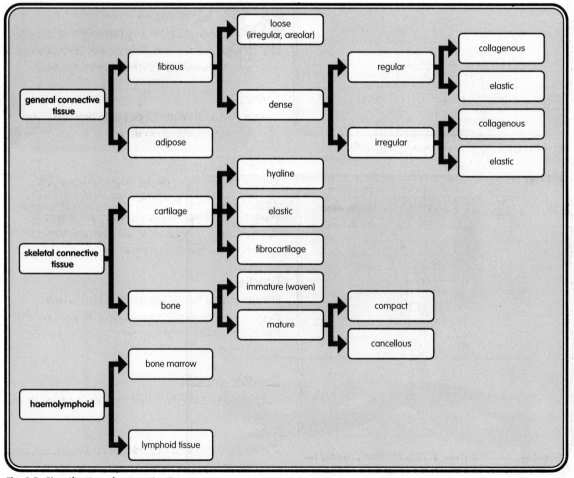

Fig. 1.5 Classification of connective tissue.

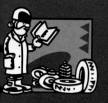

2. Muscle

OVERVIEW OF MUSCLE

Muscle is a tissue made up of contractile cells. These cells are capable of producing movement or tension. Other examples of contractile cells include myoepithelial cells (see p. 47) and myofibroblasts, found in connective tissue.

Three types of muscle tissue are found in the human body—skeletal, cardiac, and smooth (Fig. 2.1).

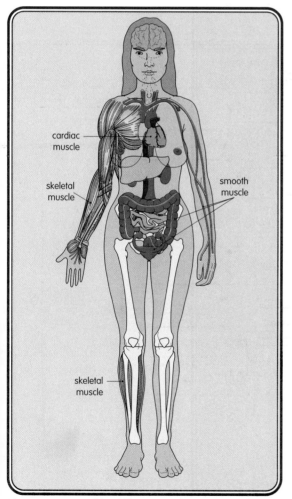

Fig. 2.1 Location of the different muscle types in the human body.

Skeletal muscle

The alternative names for skeletal muscle are striated—from its histological appearance—or voluntary—from the mechanism by which contraction is controlled.

Sites

The majority of muscle found within the body is skeletal (Fig. 2.1). It is found in the limbs, thorax, abdominal wall, pelvis, and face.

Control

Contraction of skeletal muscle tends to be voluntary or reflex and is controlled by the somatic nervous system.

Histological appearance

Skeletal muscle cells are long and thin and therefore often referred to as muscle fibres. The cells are multinucleated and appear cross-striated under light microscopy.

Cell size

Skeletal muscle cells are 50–60 µm in diameter (range 10–100 µm) and up to 10 cm long.

Nature of contraction

Rapid contraction and relaxation of skeletal muscle occurs as a twitch. The nature of the stimulus is important because, if the muscle is stimulated rapidly and repetitively, contractions may summate to produce smooth and sustained contractions.

Function

Skeletal muscle has an important role in voluntary movement of the skeleton and maintenance of posture. It is also involved in the movement of the tongue and globe of eye.

Cardiac muscle

The alternative name for cardiac muscle is myocardium.

Sites

Myocardium forms the muscular component of the heart (Fig. 2.1) lying between the pericardium and endocardium (Fig. 2.33; p. 38).

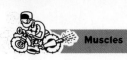

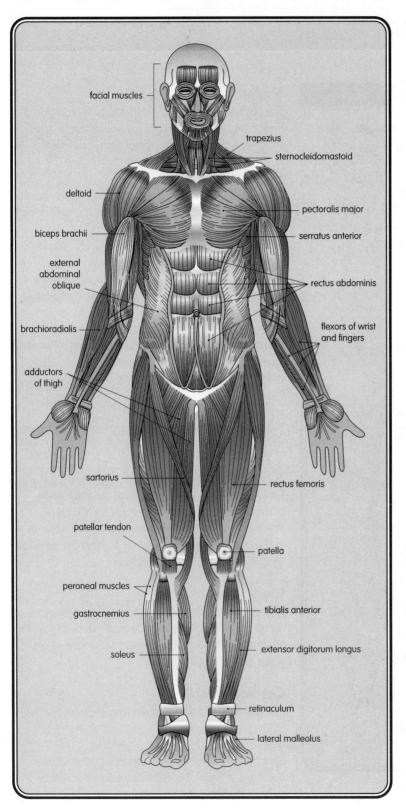

Fig. 2.2A Anterior view of major muscle groups in the body. (Courtesy of Dr K.M. Backhouse.)

facial muscles

trapezius

sternocleidomastoid

deltoid

pectoralis major

biceps brachii

serratus anterior

external abdominal oblique

rectus abdominis

brachioradialis

flexors of wrist and fingers

adductors of thigh

sartorius

rectus femoris

patellar tendon

patella

peroneal muscles

gastrocnemius

tibialis anterior

soleus

extensor digitorum longus

retinaculum

lateral malleolus

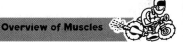

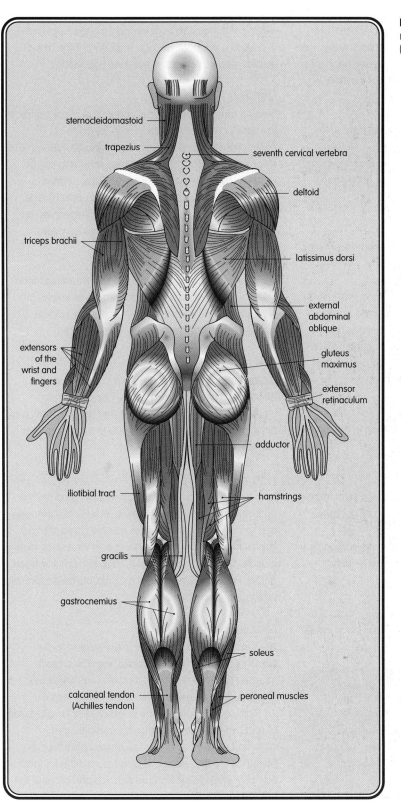

Fig. 2.2B Posterior view of major muscle groups in the body. (Courtesy of Dr K.M. Backhouse.)

sternocleidomastoid

trapezius

seventh cervical vertebra

deltoid

triceps brachii

latissimus dorsi

external abdominal oblique

extensors of the wrist and fingers

gluteus maximus

extensor retinaculum

adductor

iliotibial tract

hamstrings

gracilis

gastrocnemius

soleus

calcaneal tendon (Achilles tendon)

peroneal muscles

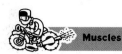

Control

Contraction of myocardium is regulated by pacemaker cells within the tissue. The autonomic nervous system can modify contraction of myocardium by altering heart rate and therefore the duration and strength of contraction.

Histological appearance

As with skeletal muscle, longitudinal and transverse striations are seen under light microscopy. However, cardiac cells are smaller and branched and have single central nuclei. Intercellular junctions are often seen. These are called intercalated discs.

Cell size

Myocardium cells are 15 μm in diameter and 100 μm long.

Nature of contraction

Myocardium undergoes spontaneous and rhythmical contractions. These contractions are always brief twitches followed by a long refractory period. This enables cardiac muscle to relax, allowing the heart to fill with blood. The long refractory period means that summation of contractions does not occur.

Function

Myocardium pumps deoxygenated blood to the lungs and oxygenated blood to the body tissues.

Smooth muscle

The alternative name for smooth muscle is involuntary muscle, from the mechanism by which contraction is controlled.

Smooth muscle can be divided into visceral (single unit or syncytial) or multi-unit types. Most smooth muscle is of the visceral type.

Sites

Single-unit smooth muscle is found in small blood vessels, the ducts of secretory glands, and the walls of hollow organs of the gastrointestinal and urogenital systems (Fig. 2.1). Multi-unit smooth muscle is found in large blood vessels, large airways, the eye, and hair follicles.

Control

Smooth muscle contraction is under involuntary control. In the case of visceral smooth muscle, initiation of contraction is inherent (pacemaker cells within the smooth muscle tissue which discharge irregularly) and can be modified by hormones, local metabolites, and the autonomic nervous system. Multi-unit smooth muscle, however, is neurogenic and initiation of contraction is under the control of the autonomic nervous system.

Histological appearance

The structure of smooth muscle is less organized than skeletal muscle and myocardium as no striations are seen under light microscopy. The cells are spindle shaped and have large, single, central nuclei.

Cell size

Smooth muscle cells are 2–10 μm in diameter and 20–400 μm long. Cell size varies, depending on location, e.g. very small cells (20 μm) are found in small blood vessels while cells up to 400 μm in length are found in the uterus.

Nature of contraction

Low-force contraction of smooth muscle occurs with relatively little energy expenditure. In the case of multi-unit smooth muscle, individual muscle fibres contract. This is the same as skeletal muscle. In visceral smooth muscle, however, as the whole muscle mass contracts and not individual muscle fibres, contraction is slow and sustained.

Function

The functions of smooth muscle are related to the structure in which they are found, e.g. the smooth muscle component of blood vessels regulates blood flow by altering the diameter of the blood vessels.

Multi-unit smooth muscle is involved in the alteration of pupil size by contraction of iris muscles, and accommodation by contraction of the ciliary muscle. Multi-unit smooth muscle is also responsible for 'goose bumps', which result from contraction of muscle at the base of each hair follicle.

> **Cardiac muscle is a type of striated muscle and its properties can be considered to lie between those of smooth and skeletal muscle.**

Skeletal and multi-unit smooth muscle may be referred to as neurogenic muscle, i.e. muscle in which contraction arises as a result of nerve stimulation.

Cardiac and visceral smooth muscle may be referred to as myogenic muscle, i.e. they require no nerve stimulation for contraction that arises from within the muscle owing to the presence of pacemaker cells.

○ Outline the differences between the three types of muscle found in the body.
○ What are the sites at which the three types of muscle are found?
○ Distinguish between neurogenic and myogenic contraction.

ORGANIZATION OF SKELETAL MUSCLE

Distribution of skeletal muscle

Contraction generated by a muscle depends on:
• The length of the muscle fibres.
• The volume/number of muscle fibres.
• The rate at which fibre length changes.

This can be illustrated by the following example. Consider two pieces of muscle tissue, of equal volume. One is long and narrow, the other short but broad in cross-section. The long muscle will allow a greater degree of shortening but, because of its narrow cross-section, it cannot generate much force of contraction. By contrast, the shorter muscle cannot contract over any great length but, because its cross-section incorporates many muscle fibres, it generates a large force of contraction.

Muscles assume a variety of shapes, depending on the type of contraction involved. For example, a multipennate arrangement results in a large number of short fibres attached to a single tendon and the force of contraction is great and concentrated on the tendon (Fig. 2.3).

Muscles are arranged in two groups:
• A functional group in which one muscle is the main

participant and the other muscles help to perform a movement: e.g. flexion at the elbow joint is due to the action of biceps with the help of brachialis, brachioradialis, and the forearm flexor muscles.
• An antagonistic group in which muscles oppose the movement of the functional group: e.g. triceps, assisted by anconeus, antagonize the action of biceps by causing extension at the elbow (Fig. 2.4).

A muscle can belong to more than one group: e.g. latissimus dorsi is involved in both adduction and extension of the shoulder joint.

Each end of a muscle is usually attached to bone. The origin, or head, is the attachment site at which there is little movement when the muscle performs its main action (see Fig. 2.4). The insertion is the more mobile attachment site.

The terms proximal attachment and distal attachment may be more appropriate as, depending on movement, the origin (proximal attachment) may be more mobile than the insertion (distal attachment).

Muscles are attached to bone by fibrous connective tissue. Examples of skeletal muscles that do not attach to bone include those of the tongue. In addition, rings of skeletal muscle or sphincters, e.g. the external urethral sphincters, that controls passage of urine from the bladder to the urethra do not attach to bone.

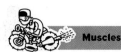

Tendon

A tendon is an inelastic, flexible cord, consisting of closely packed collagen fibres, which attaches muscle to bone.

Aponeurosis

An aponeurosis is a thin sheet of fibrous connective tissue attaching muscle to bone. It is found in muscles that have a wide attachment area to bone, e.g. the anterior abdominal wall. An aponeurosis may be considered a broad tendon.

Sesamoid bone

Sesamoid bone is a small bone found within the tendons of certain muscles, e.g. the patella and some bones in the hand and foot. Its presence may correlate with sites susceptible to wear and tear. Sesamoid bone may also provide extra leverage.

Microstructure of skeletal muscle

Arrangement of muscle tissue

Whole muscle consists of fibres which are arranged in bundles called fasciculi. Connective tissue lies between the individual muscle fibres and fasciculi. In addition there is a dense connective tissue coat surrounding the whole muscle (Fig. 2.5).

Skeletal muscle has a rich blood supply. The blood vessels and nerves divide and extend throughout the perimysium—collagen connective tissue that surrounds fasciculi.

Smaller fasciculi are found in muscles involved in fine movement; hence, the size of fasciculi is suggestive of function.

Micro-environment of skeletal muscle

Skeletal muscle fibres are arranged in parallel within a fasciculus (Fig. 2.6).

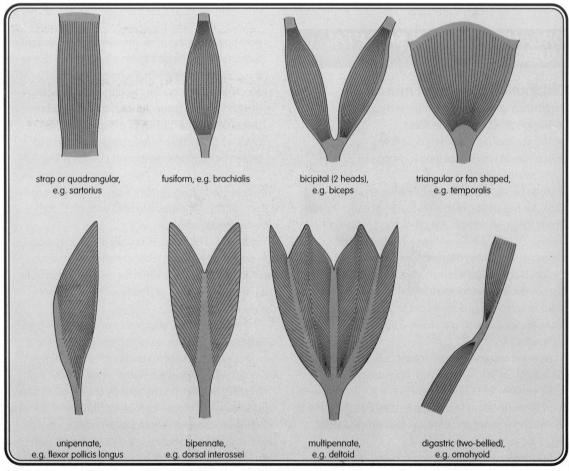

strap or quadrangular, e.g. sartorius

fusiform, e.g. brachialis

bicipital (2 heads), e.g. biceps

triangular or fan shaped, e.g. temporalis

unipennate, e.g. flexor pollicis longus

bipennate, e.g. dorsal interossei

multipennate, e.g. deltoid

digastric (two-bellied), e.g. omohyoid

Fig. 2.3 Fibre configurations and shapes of muscles in the human body.

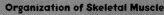

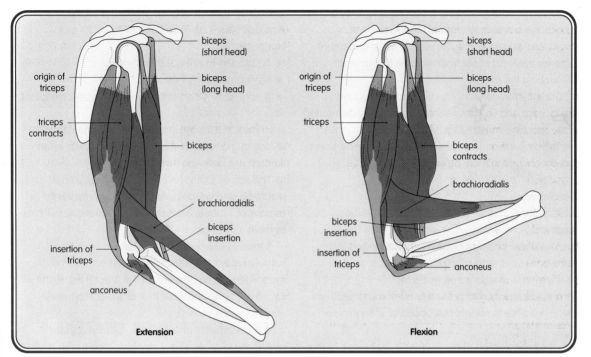

Fig. 2.4 Arrangement of muscles in antagonistic pairs demonstrated at the elbow joint.

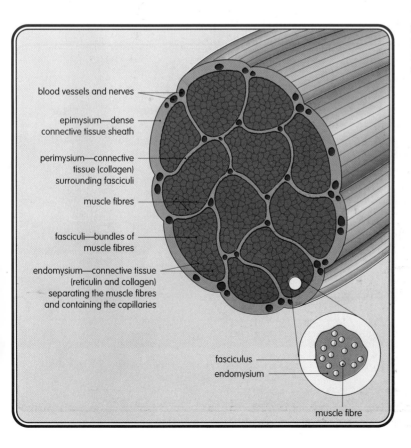

Fig. 2.5 Cross-section of whole muscle showing the arrangement of muscles into fasciculi and fibres surrounded by connective tissue.

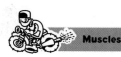

Although skeletal muscle fibres are long, they do not extend the whole length of the muscle but are organized as overlapping bundles. This arrangement enables the force of contraction to be transmitted throughout the muscle.

Skeletal muscle fibres can be divided into three types: I, IIa, and IIb. All three types are widely distributed throughout the muscle (Fig. 2.7).

The properties of the different types of muscle fibres are considered in more detail on p. 31 (Fig. 2.25).

Sarcomere

Muscle fibres, or myofibres, are cells containing myofibrils.

Myofibrils consist of myofilaments arranged in contractile units called sarcomeres.

Two types of myofilaments occur:
- Thick filaments mainly composed of myosin protein.
- Thin filaments mainly composed of actin protein.

It is the organization of myofilaments that leads to the striated appearance of muscle (Figs 2.8 and 2.9).

Cellular structure of muscle fibre

A muscle fibre is a specialized cell (Fig. 2.10) that comprises:
- A sarcolemma or cell membrane.
- Sarcoplasm or cytoplasm.
- A sarcoplasmic reticulum or endoplasmic reticulum.

Each muscle fibre cell has multiple peripheral nuclei, glycogen granules, and mitochondria that lie in the sarcoplasm between myofibrils.

The sarcoplasmic reticulum runs longitudinally along myofibrils and wraps around groups of myofibrils. In regions of T tubules, the sarcoplasmic reticulum forms terminal cisternae.

T tubules are channels that extend from the sarcolemma of the muscle fibre and surround each muscle fibre at the junction of the A and I band, the AI junction. T tubules ensure that all the sarcomeres contract synchronously.

A triad consists of a T tubule with sarcoplasmic reticulum on either side. Depolarization (p. 18) is transmitted through the T tubule, causing release of

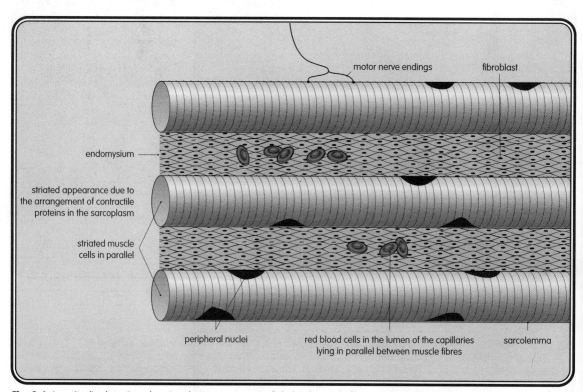

Fig. 2.6 Longitudinal section showing the arrangement of skeletal muscle fibres within a fasciculus.

Classification of different types of skeletal muscle fibres			
Fibre type	Colour	Speed and force of twitch	Resistance to fatigue
I	red (because of myoglobin)	slow, only 10% of force of type IIb	high (fatigue resistant)
IIa	intermediate	fast, but force and speed less than type IIb	intermediate (fatigue resistant)
IIb	white	fast and high force	low (fatigues after repeated stimulation), fast fatiguable

Fig. 2.7 Classification of the different types of skeletal muscle fibres.

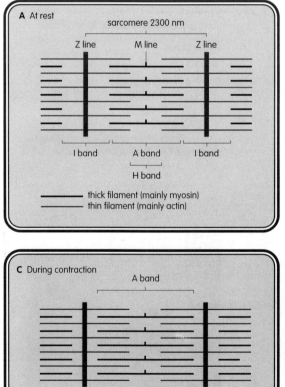

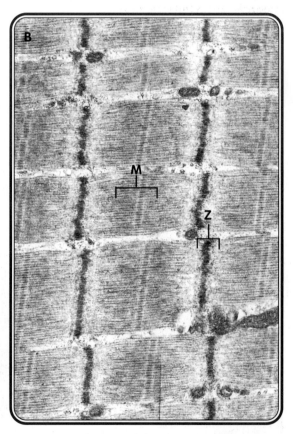

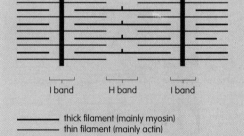

Fig. 2.8 Arrangement of contractile proteins in the sarcomere at rest and during contraction. At rest (A), the H and I bands represent areas in which the thick and thin filaments do not overlap. The Z line anchors the actin filaments and the M line anchors the myosin filaments. The pattern of actin and myosin filaments is demonstrated clearly on the electron micrograph (B). During contraction (C), the Z lines 'slide' closer together, causing shortening of muscle. The A band remains constant in width but the I and H band shorten. (M, M line; Z, Z line). (Electron micrograph courtesy of Dr T. Gray.)

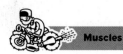
Ca^{2+} into the sarcoplasm. Ca^{2+} in the sarcoplasm triggers muscular contraction.

Replacement of muscle fibres

Satellite cells are small spindle-shaped cells that lie between the sarcolemma and basal lamina in adult skeletal muscle. These are visible with electron microscopy.

If muscle damage occurs but the basal lamina remains intact, several events occur:

- Proliferation of the satellite cells to form myoblasts.
- Fusion of myoblasts to form myotubules.
- Formation of new muscle fibres in which the nuclei are centrally, rather than peripherally, placed.

If the basal lamina becomes damaged, fibroblasts are activated and repair involves scar formation.

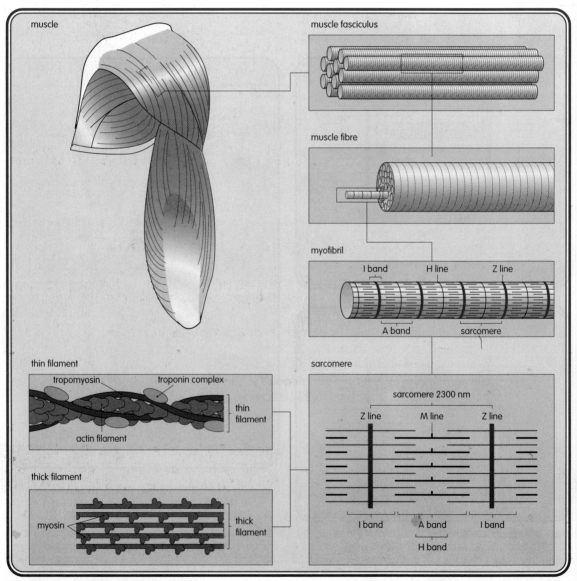

Fig. 2.9 Organization of skeletal muscle.

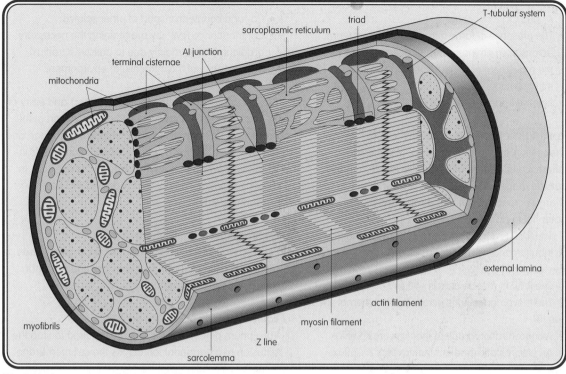

Fig. 2.10 Components of the muscle fibre.

- Describe how muscle is arranged and how shape can alter the characteristics of contraction.
- Explain the terms origin, insertion, tendon, aponeurosis, and sesamoid bone.
- Diagrammatically demonstrate the organization of skeletal muscle into fasciculi and muscle fibres.
- What is the difference between a myofibre, myofibril, and myofilament.
- Explain the term sarcomere.
- Explain the term triad in describing the cellular structure of skeletal muscle.
- Describe the role of satellite cells in adult skeletal muscle.

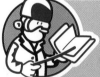

Although the overall intracellular concentration of Ca^{2+} is relatively low, remember that there is a high concentration of Ca^{2+} in the sarcoplasmic reticulum.

CELLULAR PHYSIOLOGY OF SKELETAL MUSCLE

Ion balance and the resting membrane potential

There are differences in the ionic composition of the intracellular fluid (ICF) and extracellular fluid (ECF) of muscle cells (Fig. 2.11). These are due to:

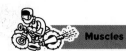
- The selective permeability of the cell membrane to K^+ and Cl^-.
- The presence of large intracellular impermeant anions from amino acid metabolism. These result in the movement of Cl^- extracellularly and K^+ intracellularly.
- Relative impermeability to Na^+.

Resting membrane potential

The resting membrane potential (RMP) is the difference in voltage between the inside and the outside of the cell at rest. This separation of charge across the cell membrane has the potential to do work.

The RMP is a result of the differences in the distribution and permeabilities of ions across the cell membrane (Fig. 2.12).

The RMP in muscle cells is −90 mV.

The movement of ions across the cell membrane is due to:

- A concentration gradient that favours K^+ efflux.
- An electrostatic gradient that favours K^+ influx.

Na^+/K^+ ATPase pump

Sites: The Na^+/K^+ ATPase pump is found in the membranes of all body cells (Fig. 2.12).

Functions: The functions of the Na^+/K^+ ATPase pump are:

Distribution of ions in the ICF and ECF of muscle cells		
Ion	**ICF (mmol/L)**	**ECF (mmol/L)**
Na^+	12	145
K^+	155	4
H^+	13×10^{-5}	3.8×10^{-5}
Ca^{2+}	8	1.5
Cl^-	3.8	12.0
HCO_3^-	8	27
A^-	155	0

Fig. 2.11 Distribution of ions in the intracellular fluid (ICF) and extracellular fluid (ECF) of muscle cells. A^-, Organic impermeant anions. (Adapted with permission from *Review of Medical Physiology* 17th edn, by W.F. Ganong, Appleton & Lange, 1995.)

- Maintenance of cell volume.
- Co- and countertransport of other solutes.
- Contribution to RMP (by maintaining the necessary gradient; RMP is mainly due to passive K^+ efflux).
- Maintenance of the intracellular environment.

Mechanism of action: The removal of $3Na^+$ and entry of $2K^+$ expends an ATP molecule. Phosphorylation of the protein subunits results in a conformational change and binding of Na^+, whereas dephosphorylation results in K^+ binding, which causes the protein to revert back to its original shape. This cycle is repeated 100 times per second (Fig. 2.12).

Electrochemical equilibrium

Electrochemical equilibrium (E) of K^+ is achieved when the forces acting in both directions are equal so that there is no net movement of K^+.

Equilibrium potential

Equilibrium potential is the voltage required to stop the diffusion of a permeant ion across the cell membrane. It can be calculated from the Nernst equation, given that the ion is permeable to the cell membrane, and assuming that the Nernst potential is the potential inside the membrane and that the potential outside the membrane is zero.

$$E_{ion} = \frac{\pm 61 \log [ion]_{ECF}}{\log [ion]_{ICF}}$$

E, equilibrium potential of the ion; 61, a constant which takes into account the valency of the ion (Z), the absolute temperature (T), the gas constant (R) and the electrical constant (F); [ion], the ion concentration in mMol/L. Note that E_K is −95 mV, which is close to the value of the RMP of a muscle cell, implying that the cell membrane is mainly permeable to K^+.

Effects of Na^+ and K^+ channels on the membrane potential

Depolarization

Depolarization results from the opening of Na^+ channels and a Na^+ influx.

The resultant membrane potential is less negative than the RMP.

Hyperpolarization

Hyperpolarization occurs upon closure of Na^+ channels and opening of K^+ channels, resulting in a K^+ efflux to

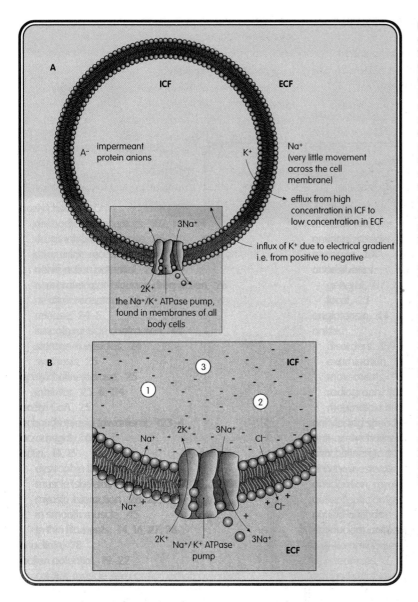

Fig. 2.12 Factors involved in the determination and maintenance of the resting membrane potential. (RMP). K^+ is the key player. (A) The Na^+ pump is found in membranes of all body cells. The mechanism of action is as follows: removal of 3 Na^+ and entry of 2 K^+, expending 1 ATP molecule; phosphorylation of the protein subunits, produces a conformational change and binding of Na^+; and dephosphorylation results in binding of K^+ and reversion of protein to original shape. The cycle is repeated 100 times per second.

Other contributors to RMP are shown in (B).
1. There is a passive leakage of a small amount of Na^+ from ECF to ICF along a concentration gradient.
2. Passive movement of Cl^- from ICF to ECF along an electrical gradient.
3. Presence of impermeant protein anions (A^-).
(Note that the bulk of the solution is electrochemically neutral. The excess ions close to the cell membrane are a small proportion. However, they are significant enough to cause movements across the cell membrane.) (ICF, intracellular fluid; ECF, extracellular fluid.)

restore normal RMP, which may be exceeded.

The resultant membrane potential is more negative than the RMP.

Action potential

An action potential (AP) is a transient depolarization of the cell membrane beyond a critical level (Fig. 2.13). When there is slow depolarization of a cell in response to a stimulus there is a 'critical level' or 'threshold' at which an AP is generated via the triggering of voltage-gated ion channels. It is an important means of transmitting information through the nervous system and initiating contraction of muscle cells.

The size and duration of the AP within different cell types is variable.

Initiation of the AP

APs are usually initiated:

- At synapses—specialized junctions between cells.
- By the passage of current from one cell to another via gap junctions.

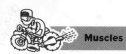

Either of these result in a slow depolarization of the cell membrane.

Threshold is the critical level of depolarization at which an AP is initiated.

The **all-or-none law** states that, once an AP has been initiated the size is constant for a given type of cell and that altering the stimulus strength does not affect this.

Ionic basis of the AP

Na⁺ and K⁺ movements across the cell membrane are important (Fig. 2.14).

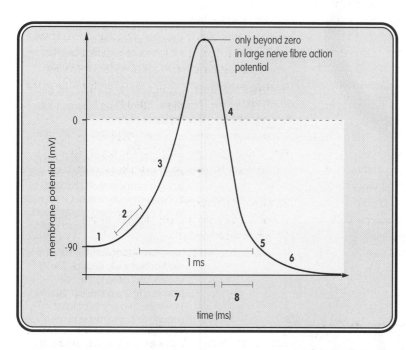

Fig. 2.13 *Phases of the action potential (AP). (1) resting membrane potential; (2) initial slow depolarization of cell in response to stimulus; (3) opening of voltage-gated Na⁺ channels when threshold is reached; (4) repolarization, i.e. opening of voltage-gated K⁺ channels; (5) return to resting membrane potential (−90 mV) (6) hyperpolarization due to 'excessive' K⁺ efflux; (7) absolute refractory period (AP may not be initiated); (8) relative refractory period (greater stimulus than normal to initiate the AP).*

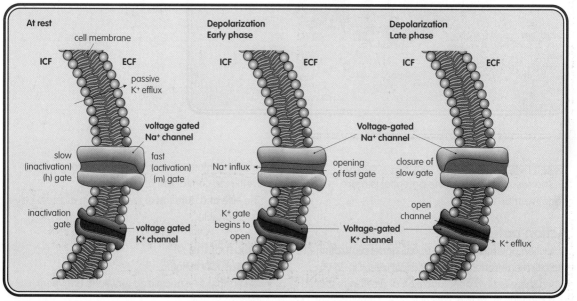

Fig. 2.14 Changes in voltage-activated channels during an action potential derived from studies using the voltage clamp and selective channel blockers. (ICF, intracellular fluid; ECF, extracellular fluid.)

At rest, both voltage-activated Na$^+$ and K$^+$ channels are 'closed'. K$^+$ moves passively along a concentration gradient out of the cell.

Early phase of depolarization

During the early phase of depolarization, the fast gate (m-gate) of a voltage-gated Na$^+$ channel opens and the slow gate (h-gate) starts to close. As the slow gate takes longer to close, there is an influx of Na$^+$. This influx results in the activation of more Na$^+$ channels via a feedback mechanism.

The voltage-activated K$^+$ channel starts to open slowly.

Late phase of depolarization

During the late phase of depolarization, the slow gate of a voltage-gated Na$^+$ channel is closed and there is no more influx of Na$^+$. The slow gate re-opens when \RMP is reached, i.e. when the fast gate is closed.

The K$^+$ channel is open and remains so until RMP is restored. Closure of the channel is slow, and hyperpolarization may occur following an AP.

Propagation of the AP

An AP occurring at any one site on the cell membrane causes changes in the adjacent parts of the membrane, allowing propagation of the AP. This can be explained by the **local circuit theory** (Fig. 2.15). Propagation can occur in both directions.

Saltatory conduction

Saltatory conduction occurs in myelinated nerve fibres (Fig. 2.16). The local circuit theory still applies but the current can leave the axon only at nodes of Ranvier. This results in a greater conduction velocity because the current density at the nodes is greater, so depolarization is more rapid.

The circuit of current can travel a number of internodal lengths and still be able to depolarize a node to threshold. This produces a large safety factor.

Conduction velocity

In nerves the conduction velocity (CV) ranges from 100 m/s to less than 1 m/s.

Factors affecting conduction velocity are:

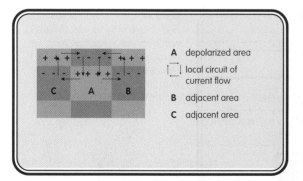

Fig. 2.15 Local circuit theory. The local circuit of current may cause sufficient depolarization in B and/or C to initiate an action potential. This can then be propagated in the same way.

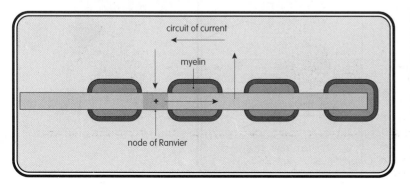

Fig. 2.16 Saltatory conduction in myelinated nerve fibres. The current is only able to leave at the nodes of ranvier. In this way, the circuit of current can be thought of as 'jumping' from node to node, allowing a greater speed of conduction.

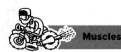

- Fibre diameter, i.e. myelin sheath, large nerve fibres—increasing the fibre diameter increases the conduction velocity.
- Temperature—increasing temperature increases the conduction velocity. However, above 40°C the conduction velocity decreases until there is 'heat block'.
- Strength of local circuits—stronger local circuits result in a greater conduction velocity.

The synapse

The junction at which nerve cells communicate with each other is called a synapse.

Synapses can be electrical, i.e. direct transmission of current from presynaptic cell to target cell through ion channels, or chemical, i.e. release of a chemical that binds to protein receptors on the target cell membrane, causing direct or indirect opening of ion channels (Fig. 2.17).

Transmission of a signal at a chemical synapse involves:

- An AP propagated at the nerve terminal.
- Depolarization of the nerve terminal.
- Voltage-activated Ca^{2+} channels open, causing an influx of Ca^{2+}.
- Vesicles in the active zone fusing with the presynaptic membrane. Neurotransmitter is released by exocytosis.

The main ion responsible for the RMP is K^+. However the RMP is not equal to the equilibrium potential of potassium (E_K) owing to:

- Small concentration of Na^+ leaking from E_{CF} to I_{CF}.
- Diffusion of Cl^-.
- Presence of protein impermeant ions (A^-).
- The activities of the Na^+/K^+ pump.

Comparison of electrical and chemical synapses		
Property	**Electrical**	**Chemical**
site	nerves, heart, smooth muscle, liver, epithelium	most of synapses in body, including skeletal muscle and brain
structures seen at synapse	gap junctions	presynaptic vesicles and mitochondria, postsynaptic receptors
mechanism of transmission	ionic current	chemical messenger
cytoplasmic continuity between presynaptic and postsynaptic cell	yes	no
synaptic cleft	3.5 nm	20–40 nm
nature of transmission	rapid, usually excitatory effect on target cell	synaptic delay 1–5 ms, excitatory or inhibitory effect on target cell
plasticity	no	yes
amplification of signal	no	yes

Fig. 2.17 Comparison of electrical and chemical synapses. (Adapted with permission from *Human Physiology and Mechanisms of Disease* 8th edn, by A.C. Guyton, W.B. Saunders, 1991.)

- The neurotransmitter binding to protein receptors in the postsynaptic membrane.
- Changes in the postsynaptic membrane, leading to depolarization or hyperpolarization of the target cell.

Transmission of a signal at an electrical synapse involves:
- Depolarization of the presynaptic membrane.
- Direct flow of current through gap-junction ion channels to target cell.
- Depolarization of the target cell.

Local anaesthetics
Local anaesthetics are drugs that are used to provide temporary relief of pain. They are weak bases; 90% are un-ionized and can cross the cell membrane but are not very effective at blocking the Na^+ channels, while 10% are ionized and block the Na^+ channels from inside the axon when the channels are open.

The more common local anaesthetics include lignocaine, bupivicaine, prilocaine, benzocaine, and cocaine.

Vasoconstrictors (e.g. adrenaline) are often administered with local anaesthetics. The constricted blood vessels prevent too much local anaesthetic diffusing away from the relevant site. This results in a longer duration of action and lower chance of systemic toxicity.

Vasoconstrictors are never used in sites with small blood vessels (e.g. fingers, ears), owing to the risk of ischaemia resulting from vasospasm.

Mechanism of action: Local anaesthetics block Na^+ channels thereby preventing depolarization and propagation of APs. The un-ionized form crosses the cell membrane and 10% ionizes in the cytoplasm. This ionized form then blocks open Na^+ channels from within. Nerve fibres with a small diameter are more affected; hence, local anaesthetics can block the sensation of pain without affecting touch.

Use dependency: The more a nerve is stimulated the greater the block achieved, as the Na^+ channels are blocked when open.

Adverse effects: Local anaesthetics can affect the cardiovascular system, by causing hypotension or cardiac arrest, or the central nervous system (CNS) by causing restlessness, sleepiness, convulsions, and respiratory depression. Anaphylaxis can also occur.

Neuromuscular junction
Structure of the neuromuscular junction
At the neuromuscular junction (NMJ, Fig. 2.18) each muscle fibre is innervated by one motor nerve.

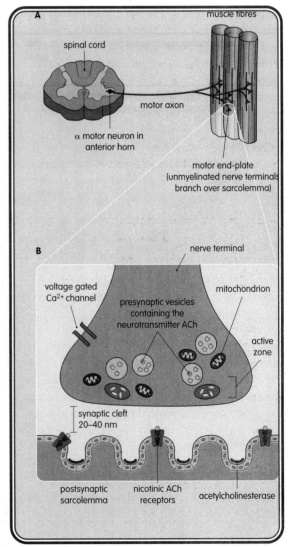

Fig. 2.18 Diagram demonstrating (A) the motor end-plate and (B) the structure of the neuromuscular junction at a chemical synapse. (ACh, acetylcholine.)

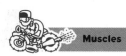

The nerve terminal invaginates into the muscle fibre near its midpoint to form a depression in the muscle membrane, termed the synaptic trough (gutter). However, the nerve terminal does not cross the muscle membrane.

The synaptic cleft is:
- The space between the nerve terminal and the muscle membrane.
- Occupied by connective tissue and ECF.

Presynaptic nerve terminal

Vesicles
At the presynaptic nerve terminal, acetylcholine (ACh) is synthesized in the cytoplasm and then stored in vesicles (about 10 000 molecules per vesicle) with an ATP molecule. At rest, 85% of ACh is stored in the vesicles and 15% is present in the cytoplasm.

Mitochondria
Numerous mitochondria provide energy for the uptake of choline and synthesis of ACh.

Active zones
Active zones are specialized regions of the presynaptic membrane. They are sites of neurotransmitter release and are positioned so they lie opposite a junctional fold in the postsynaptic membrane.

Voltage-activated Ca^{2+} channels
Voltage-activated Ca^{2+} channels are believed to be adjacent to active zones. The channels open in response to an AP. The associated influx of Ca^{2+} causes the vesicles to move to the active zone.

Postsynaptic membrane

Motor end-plate
The motor end-plate is a specialized region of the muscle fibre membrane at which the terminal branches of the motor nerve communicate with the muscle fibre.

Junctional folds
Junctional folds are folds in the motor end-plate upon which nicotinic ACh receptors (nicAChR) are located. These folds increase the surface area upon which the transmitter can act.

Basal lamina
The basal lamina is connective tissue lying between the nerve terminal and muscle fibre

membrane. Large quantities of the enzyme acetylcholinesterase are found here, particularly at the bases of the junctional folds.

Nicotinic ACh receptor
The nicotinic ACh receptor (nicAChR) consists of five protein subunits (2α, 1β, 1γ, and 1δ). The binding of two ACh molecules (one to each of the two α subunits) induces a conformational change and the channel opens. The channel is permeable to both K^+ and Na^+. However, concentration gradients favour Na^+ influx.

When a nerve AP arrives at the NMJ a sequence of events, lasting 10–15 ms, takes place. This sequence is numbered to correspond to Fig. 2.19, as follows:

1. The AP arrives at the nerve terminal.
2. The voltage-activated Ca^{2+} channels open, allowing Ca^{2+} influx.
3. Ca^{2+} influx attracts presynaptic vesicles to the active zones.
4. Vesicles fuse to the presynaptic membrane and release ACh in 'packets' by the process of exocytosis.
5. ACh diffuses across the synaptic cleft to bind to nicAChR on the junctional folds. There is activation of channels and an influx of Na^+ occurs.
6. Na^+ influx depolarizes the muscle. This is called an end-plate potential (e.p.p.). The end-plate potential

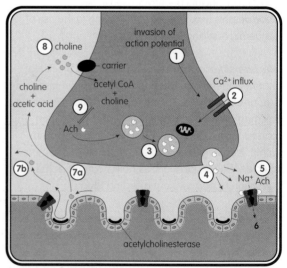

Fig. 2.19 Events at the neuromuscular junction upon arrival of a nerve action potential. Refer to text for an explanation of the sequence (this occurs in 10–15 ms). (ACh, acetylcholine.)

depolarizes adjacent regions of the muscle membrane. Upon reaching threshold, an AP occurs in the muscle fibre.

7. Rapid removal of ACh from the synaptic trough terminates the activation of the receptors. This removal occurs in two ways: (A) by the action of acetylcholinesterase, which hydrolyses ACh to choline and acetic acid; (B) a small amount that has diffused out of the trough is broken down by pseudocholinesterase in the plasma.

8. Uptake of choline into nerve terminals is the rate-limiting step of ACh synthesis. This is an active process requiring the hydrolysis of ATP, and involves two carrier systems—the high affinity–low capacity mechanism, which is responsible for 90% of uptake, and the low affinity–high capacity mechanism.

9. Recycled choline reacts with acetyl CoA (formed in the mitochondria and transported into the cytoplasm). The enzyme choline acetyltransferase catalyses the reaction. The vesicle membrane is also recycled by endocytosis from the nerve terminal membrane. ACh is again stored in 'packets' in the nerve terminal.

AP in skeletal muscle

The ionic basis of the AP in skeletal muscle is the same as the AP in nerves. However, there are certain differences between the two (Fig. 2.20).

Drugs acting at the NMJ
Drugs acting presynaptically

Hemicholinium acts presynaptically at the NMJ by blocking the uptake of choline. There is a slow depletion of ACh in the nerve terminal.

Aminoglycosides and botulinum toxin inhibit ACh release.

Drugs enhancing transmission

Anticholinesterases enhance transmission at the NMJ by increasing the time that ACh is present in the synaptic cleft.

Mechanism of action: Anticholinesterases inhibit acetylcholinesterase. There are three main types of anticholinesterases: short-acting (up to 15 minutes) drugs such as edrophonium (these bind reversibly to the active site of the enzyme); intermediate-acting drugs, e.g. pyridostigmine and neostigmine (these bind covalently to the enzyme); and long-acting drugs, e.g. organophosphorous compounds (these form strong covalent bonds with the active site; they are often referred to as irreversible, as the enzyme is inactivated for a long period of time; they have no clinical use, but are used in chemical weapons).

Indications: Edrophonium assists in the diagnosis of myasthenia gravis. An intravenous injection leads to short-term improvement in muscle strength. Treatment involves the use of intermediate-acting anticholinesterases. Anticholinesterases reverse competitive neuromuscular block after surgery.

Adverse effects: Side effects of anticholinesterases include: paradoxical depolarizing neuromuscular block; convulsions, coma, and respiratory arrest if a lipid-soluble anticholinesterase (e.g. physostigmine) is used; and symptoms associated with the parasympathetic nervous system, as ACh is the

Comparison of the action potential of skeletal muscle with nerve		
Property	**Skeletal muscle AP**	**Nerve AP**
RMP	−80 to −90 mV	−40 mV (small nerves) to −90 mV (large nerves)
duration	1–5 ms	<1 ms
spread of AP to interior	T-tubule system	depolarization of membrane is sufficient
conduction velocity	3–5 m/s	<1–100 ms, depends on a number of factors (see page 22)

Fig. 2.20 Comparison of the action potential (AP) in skeletal muscle with that in nerves.

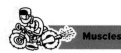

neurotransmitter acting on muscarinic receptors.

Drugs acting postsynaptically
Neuromuscular-blocking drugs are either competitive or depolarizing.

Competitive drugs
Tubocurarine and gallamine are examples of competitive neuromuscular-blocking drugs.

Mechanism of action: Neuromuscular-blocking drugs compete with ACh for binding sites on the ACh receptor in the postsynaptic membrane. There is no opening of the ion channel when they bind; therefore AP generation in muscle is less likely. Their action is reversed by anticholinesterases and enhanced by general anaesthetics.

Indications: Neuromuscular-blocking drugs are used in surgery to relax skeletal muscles, and for electroconvulsive therapy.

Adverse effects: Side effects of neuromuscular-blocking drugs include a decrease in blood pressure due to blockage of autonomic nicotinic receptors, and anaphylaxis.

Depolarizing drugs
Suxamethonium is an example of a depolarizing drug.

Mechanism of action: Depolarizing drugs are nicotinic agonists with blockage occurring due to prolonged membrane depolarization and desensitization of nicotinic receptors. Their action is potentiated by anticholinesterases.

Indications: Depolarizing drugs are used in surgery to relax skeletal muscles, and for electroconvulsive therapy. Although competitive blockers are more widely used, depolarizing drugs tend to be used for brief procedures.

Adverse effects: As initial stimulation occurs before blockage, asynchronous muscle fibre twitches may result in muscle pains following the use of depolarizing drugs. Other side effects include bradycardia due to action on muscarinic receptors.

Excitation–contraction coupling
Excitation–contraction coupling refers to the events that occur from initiation of an AP in the sarcolemma, contraction of muscle, and subsequent relaxation.

Initiation of an AP in muscle fibre
The end-plate potential (e.p.p.) resulting from a single neuronal AP is usually greater in amplitude than that required to initiate an AP in muscle fibre. For this reason the NMJ is said to have a very high '**safety factor**'.

Propagation of an AP into muscle fibre via T tubules
An AP is propagated into muscle fibre via T tubules in a sequence of events (the following numbers refer to Fig. 2.21).
1. Bidirectional propagation of the AP occurs along the sarcolemma. This causes excitation of muscle fibre along its whole length so that all sarcomeres contract simultaneously.
2. The AP is then propagated into the muscle fibre via the T tubule. There are two T tubules per sarcomere. These encircle the myofibril at the AI junction. T tubules communicate with the extracellular space.
3. The sarcoplasmic reticulum on both sides of the T tubule communicates with the T tubule via junctional feet. Depolarization of the T tubule results in a signal from the T tubule to the sarcoplasmic reticulum terminal cisternae.
4. Ca^{2+} channels then open in the sarcoplasmic reticulum and Ca^{2+} moves along a concentration gradient into the sarcoplasm around the myofibrils.

Muscle contraction
Two types of molecule—thick and thin filaments—are involved in the muscle contraction (Fig. 2.22).

Thick filament
Myosin: This is the main component of thick filament. It is a much larger protein than actin and consists of a tail, neck, and head (cross bridge) region.
   The head region possesses ATPase activity and can attach to specific binding sites on the actin molecule; the neck region is flexible, which is necessary for attachment and detachment to the actin filament, and the tail region provides strength.

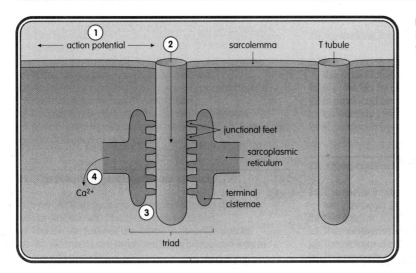

Fig. 2.21 Sarcoplasmic release of intracellular Ca^{2+}. The numbers refer to the text.

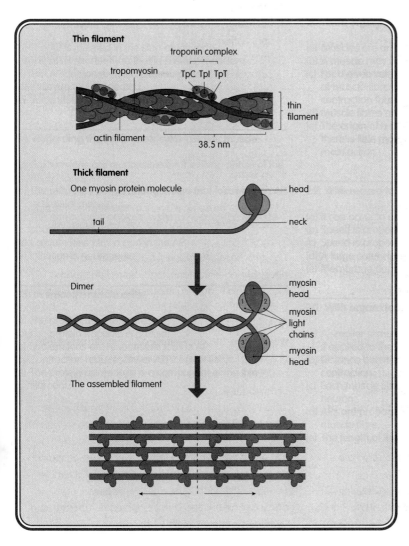

Fig. 2.22 Arrangement of contractile proteins in thin filament and thick (myosin) filament .

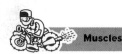

Thin filament
Actin: This is the main component of thin filament. It is capable of binding five other proteins.

Tropomyosin: This is a structural protein found bound to actin filaments. Each tropomyosin is bound to seven actin filaments.

Tropomyosin 'covers' the myosin-binding sites on the actin filament, thereby preventing a myosin–actin interaction.

Troponin: This protein consists of a complex of three subunits: T, which binds one tropomyosin, C, which has a high affinity for Ca^{2+}, and I, which has a high affinity for actin (hence the attachment of tropomyosin to actin).

The binding of Ca^{2+} causes a change in shape and movement of the associated tropomyosin. This uncovers the myosin-attachment site on actin.

α Actinin: This protein is found in the Z band.

Mechanism of contraction
Huxley's cross-bridge cycle
Huxley's cross-bridge cycle demonstrates the shortening of the sarcomere due to sliding of the actin filaments. The numbers correspond to Fig. 2.23, as follows:
1. In the resting state the myosin-attachment sites on the actin molecule are covered by tropomyosin.
2. An increase in intracellular Ca^{2+} results in the binding of Ca^{2+} to troponin C. The binding of Ca^{2+} causes a conformational change in the troponin complex, resulting in movement of the tropomyosin and uncovering of the myosin-binding sites.
3. The myosin head attaches to an actin molecule and releases the phosphate group.
4. This attachment causes the myosin head to tilt towards its tail, thereby pulling the actin filament in that direction. Tilting of the head causes release of ADP.
5. A molecule of ATP binds to the myosin head. This causes detachment of the head from the actin.
6. The ATPase action of the myosin head cleaves ATP, resulting in a myosin head with attached ADP and phosphate. The energy derived from this process

causes untilting of the head, preparing it for reattachment.

The whole process is repeated. In this way the myosin head 'walks' along the actin filament. This is the basis of the 'walk along' theory.

Relaxation of muscle
Relaxation of muscle is Ca^{2+} dependent. Upon repolarization of the muscle fibre, Ca^{2+} is actively pumped back into the sarcoplasmic reticulum. The concentration of Ca^{2+} drops and it is no longer bound to troponin.

The myosin-binding sites become 'covered' by tropomyosin again, preventing further 'walking'.

Bioenergetics of muscle contraction
Muscle contraction results in energy expenditure during:
- Interaction of actin and myosin filaments during contraction.
- Pumping of Ca^{2+} from the sarcoplasm back into the sarcoplasmic reticulum after contraction.
- Restoration of the intracellular ionic environment after muscle contraction, due to the actions of the Na^+/K^+ pump.

Sources of energy
Short term
Sarcoplasm: ATP molecules are present in sarcoplasm. These would be expended within the first 2 seconds of contraction if they were not replaced.

Creatine phosphokinase: As a substrate, creatine phosphokinase contains high-energy phosphate bonds, which can be used to phosphorylate ADP to ATP by the enzyme creatine kinase. It is located in the Z line.

Myokinase: The enzyme myokinase catalyses the transfer of a phosphate group from one ADP molecule to another to form ATP and the by-product AMP.

Intermediate term
Anaerobic glycolysis: This causes the breakdown of glucose to lactate and pyruvate with the release of energy, which is used to convert ADP to ATP. ATP is generated at double the rate of oxidative phosphorylation. See *Crash Course: Metabolism and Nutrition* for more detail.

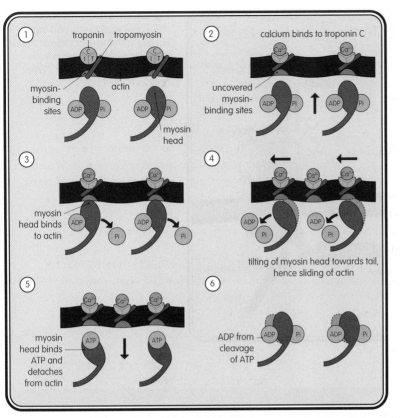

Fig. 2.23 Interaction of myosin heads with thin filaments during contraction. The numbers refer to the text.

Anaerobic glycolysis is predominant in type II muscle fibres, which have few mitochondria but many glycogen granules.

This is an intermediate-term source of energy only, as lactate and pyruvate accumulate in the cell.

Long term

Oxidative phosphorylation: This is an aerobic process in which ATP is liberated from fats, carbohydrates, and protein. See *Crash Course: Metabolism and Nutrition* for more information.

Energy can be provided for longer periods (a few hours) than with glycolysis.

Type I muscle fibres are suited to oxidative phosphorylation as they have numerous mitochondria and lipid droplets.

Myofibre cytoskeleton

The myofibre cytoskeleton is essential to the mechanical stability and function of muscle. The proteins present in the myofibre cytoskeleton are dystrophin and bridging glycoproteins.

Actin filaments are linked to dystrophin, which in turn is linked to a number of glycoproteins that extend to the

All sarcomeres in a muscle fibre contract at the same time, otherwise shortening of one sarcomere would result in lengthening of adjacent sarcomeres.

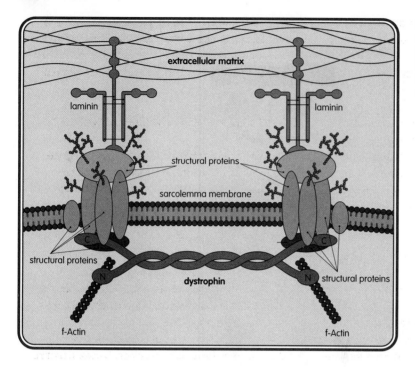

Fig. 2.24 Components of the myofibre cytoskeleton and their linkage with the extracellular matrix. (Adapted with permission from *Muscle and Nerve*, by Jah, Wiley and Sons 1994.)

- Describe the ionic composition of the ICF and ECF in muscle fibres.
- What is the difference between the RMP and the equilibrium potential?
- What is the ionic basis of an AP (demonstrate on a diagram)? Describe its initiation and propagation.
- Explain the following terms: all-or-none law, local circuit theory, and safety factor associated with saltatory conduction.
- With regard to the NMJ, describe the events that occur upon arrival of an AP at the nerve terminal to initiation of an AP in the muscle fibre.
- Describe the synthesis, storage, and breakdown of ACh.
- What are the types of drugs acting at the NMJ?
- Describe Huxley's cross-bridge cycle and the role of ATP.
- Describe the role of dystrophin protein.

surface of the sarcolemma. These glycoproteins link to laminin in the basement membrane (Fig. 2.24).

The myofibre cytoskeleton forms a link between the inside of the cell and the extracellular matrix. (The extracellular matrix supports the muscle fibre, decreasing the likelihood of tearing upon contraction.) Duchenne muscular dystrophy is an example of a condition resulting from abnormalities in the myofibre cytoskeleton (see pg 115).

FUNCTIONS OF SKELETAL MUSCLE

Motor unit

The motor unit refers to the motor neuron and all the muscle fibres innervated by it.

Each motor neuron may innervate many muscle fibres but a single muscle fibre receives input from only one motor neuron.

The number of muscle fibres innervated by a motor neuron is known as the innervation ratio. A smaller number of muscle fibres per motor neuron are present in muscles involved in fine, precise movements, e.g. ocular muscles, while a larger number are seen in muscles involved in gross movements, e.g. maintaining posture.

The muscle fibres innervated by a single motor neuron are spread out within the muscle.

The muscle fibres within a motor unit are of the same type and contract simultaneously.

There are three different types of motor units (Fig. 2.25).

Orderly recruitment

Small motor neurons innervate slow muscle fibres (type I) whereas fast muscle fibres (types IIa and IIb) are innervated by larger motor neurons. This is referred to as the **size principle**.

Smaller motor neurons require a smaller excitatory input for activation. During reflex or voluntary movement for a given excitatory input, it is the slow units that are activated first. This results in an orderly recruitment of muscle fibres, with activation of slow units first followed by fast fatigue-resistant units and finally fast fatiguable units first followed by fast fatigue-resistant units and finally fast fatiguable units. This is important *in vivo* as it allows movement to be graded by altering the level of excitatory input rather than having to select different fibre types.

Effects of denervation and reinnervation on motor units

Denervation of a motor unit results in atrophy of the muscle fibres within that unit. There may also be fibrillations on the electromyogram, shown as fine, irregular contractions of individual fibres, and an increase in sensitivity to circulating ACh.

Clinically, the signs of a lower motor neuron lesion are seen. These include a decrease in muscle tone, decrease in power, and diminished reflexes.

Some of the muscle fibres are replaced by fibrous and fatty tissue. However, this fibrous tissue shortens and contractures may form.

Other muscle fibres may be reinnervated by collaterals from the remaining adjacent motor neurons. This results in:
- Possible alteration of the fibre type, as it is the motor neuron that determines the fibre type. In

Properties of different motor unit types			
Property	**Motor unit type**		
	slow, resistant to fatigue	**fast, non-fatiguable**	**fast, fatiguable**
fibre diameter	small (type I)	intermediate (type IIa)	large (type IIb)
force of contraction	low	intermediate	high
myosin–ATPase activity (indicates rate of ATP hydrolysis and therefore speed of twitch)	low	low	high
source of energy	oxidative phosphorylation	oxidative phosphorylation and some anaerobic glycolysis	anaerobic glycolysis
glycogen content	low	intermediate	high
mitochondria	many	many	few
capillaries	many	many	few
function	fine movement and maintenance of posture	sustained activity	brief strong contractions, e.g. jumping

Fig. 2.25 Properties of different motor unit types.

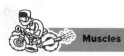
this way there may be areas of muscle containing fibres of only one type. This is termed fibre clumping and produces characteristic waveforms on a diagnostic electromyogram (EMG).
- Larger motor units.

Muscle mechanics
Isometric contraction
Isometric contraction occurs in muscle with a constant length.

Isometric tests can be used to compare force against duration of contraction of different muscles (Figs 2.26 and 2.27).

Isotonic contraction
Isotonic contraction occurs in muscle with a constant tension. The length of the muscle changes while maintaining constant tension.

Isotonic tests can be used to compare the speed of shortening of different muscle types (Fig. 2.27).

Sarcoplasmic Ca^{2+} concentration and muscle twitch
Every AP in skeletal muscle results in a similar amount of Ca^{2+} release. Hence, under isometric conditions, the force of the twitch resulting from a single AP will remain the same.

Unlike myocardium, the strength of contraction in skeletal muscle is not dependent on sarcoplasmic Ca^{2+}

concentration as each AP results in sufficient Ca^{2+} release to produce the maximal response.

Maximal response in skeletal muscle, however, is not seen with a single AP because:
- Series elasticity occurs whereby structural components (e.g. tendons, cross bridges) of the muscle are elastic and lengthen when force is generated; therefore initial shortening of muscle is slow.
- Sarcoplasmic Ca^{2+} is rapidly pumped back into the sarcoplasmic reticulum following an AP, thereby ending the response.

Force of contraction in skeletal muscle may be increased by maintaining the sarcoplasmic Ca^{2+} concentration by repetitive stimulation. This would result in greater shortening as the initial twitch would be involved in stretching of the elastic elements with no 'wasting' of force upon subsequent twitches as the elastic elements are already stretched (Fig. 2.28).

Maintained muscle contractions
Twitch
Twitch is a single contraction resulting from a single AP. It is a submaximal response.

Unfused tetanus
Unfused tetanus occurs when muscle is repetitively stimulated such that there is insufficient time for

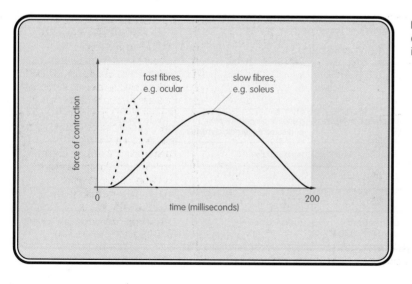

Fig. 2.26 Duration of contraction in different muscles demonstrated by isometric tests.

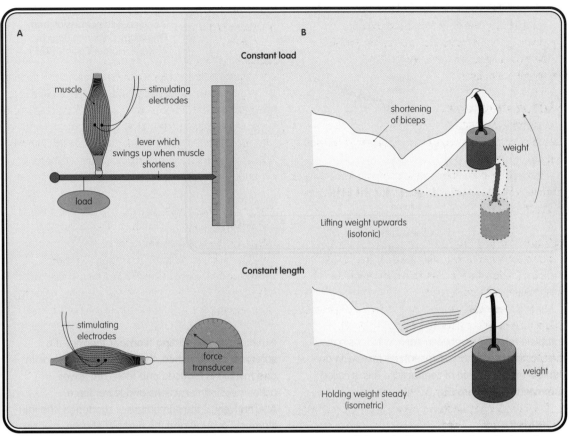

Fig. 2.27 (A) Measurement of isotonic and isometric contractions. (Modified from *Human Physiology and Mechanisms of Disease,* 8th edn by Dr A.C. Guyton, W.B. Saunders, 1992.) (B) Situations involving isotonic and isometric contractions. (Adapted with permission from *Review of Medical Physiology* ,17th edn by W.F. Ganong, Appleton Lange, 1995.)

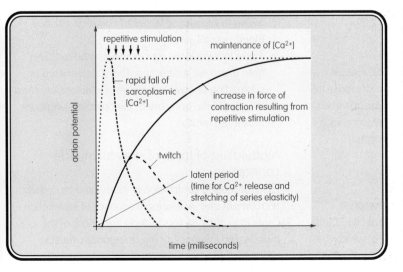

Fig. 2.28 Relationship of sarcoplasmic [Ca^{2+}] to force of contraction in skeletal muscle. Repeat stimulation results in maintenance of intracellular [Ca^{2+}]. Series elasticity refers to the inherent elasticity of muscle tissue, including its non-contractile C/T matrix. The latent period can be thought of as 'taking up the slack' before contraction of the tissue begins. In repetitive stimulation the elastic elements remain stretched, improving muscle efficiency. (Adapted with permission from *Physiology 3e*, by R.M. Berne and M.N. Levy. Mosby Year Book, 1993.)

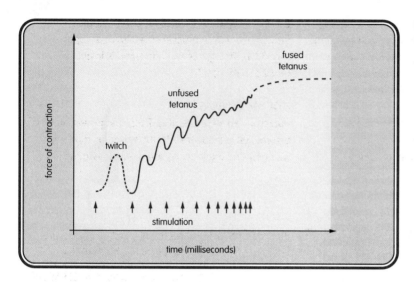

Fig. 2.29 Summation of twitches. (Adapted with permission from *Physiology Colouring Book* by W. Kapit, Harper Collins, 1987.)

complete relaxation between each twitch. As a result, the successive mechanical responses fuse, with an additive effect on force of contraction. This is called summation of twitches (Fig. 2.29).

Fused tetanus

Fused tetanus results from summation of twitches. However, there is no relaxation of muscle between each stimulus, resulting in fusion of consecutive twitches and a smooth sustained contraction.

Summation of twitches is an important means of varying the force of contraction. Therefore increasing the frequency of stimulation is an important means of modulating force of contraction (see Fig. 2.29).

Tetany

Tetany is spasm and twitching of skeletal muscle due to low levels of extracellular Ca^{2+}. A decrease in extracellular Ca^{2+} lowers the threshold for activation of muscle and nerve cells. This is not the same as a tetanus, which is a normal feature of skeletal muscle.

Length–tension relationship

The force or tension a muscle fibre generates depends on the length of the sarcomere (Fig. 2.30). There is an optimum range of lengths at which the force generated is maximum. This can be

explained by the **sliding filament theory**—if a sarcomere is stretched, the overlap between actin and myosin is reduced and there are fewer actin–myosin interactions and lower force. Alternatively, if the sarcomere is shortened, the thin filaments overlap and the number of actin–myosin interactions are again reduced.

In a whole muscle the total tension developed is the sum of active tension and passive tension.

- Total tension results from isometric contraction of muscle in response to a maximal stimulus.
- Passive tension results from stretching of the muscle in the absence of contraction and occurs owing to the elastic forces of connective tissue, blood vessels, etc.
- Active tension is the increase in tension resulting from muscular contraction. This is determined by subtracting passive tension from total tension. Most muscles in the body are at the optimum length for maximum tension.

Modulation of force of skeletal muscle contraction

Force of muscle contraction is modulated by orderly recruitment and increasing frequency of stimulation. Other important factors include the length of the muscle and influence of the antagonistic muscle groups.

Force–velocity relationship

The force–velocity relationship is found by stimulating a muscle under isotonic conditions and measuring the speed of shortening with different loads. The speed of shortening is decreased with increasing loads (Fig. 2.31A)

Speed of shortening varies with different fibre types. This occurs owing to the existence of myosin isoforms. In fast fibres, myosin ATPase activity is rapid and therefore cross-bridge cycling and shortening of muscle fibres is more rapid (Fig. 2.31). The speed of shortening is inversely related to the load.

Power curves

Power = velocity × load (Fig. 2.32). The power of muscle contraction is influenced by the speed of shortening (velocity) and the load. Although increasing the load

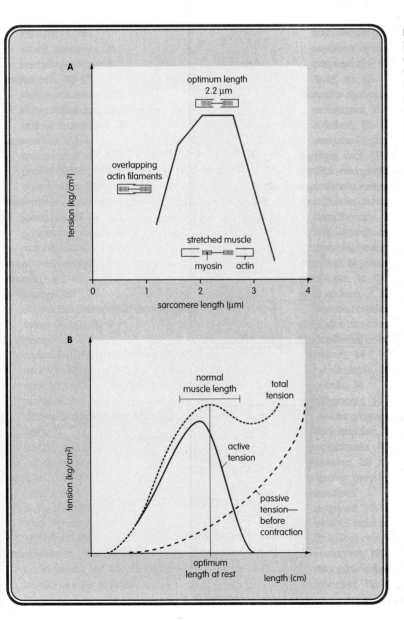

Fig. 2.30 (A) Effect of sarcomere length on the active tension developed by an individual muscle fibre upon contraction. (B) Effect of muscle length on tension. Increasing the passive tension initially increases the total tension. Further increases in passive tension lead to a decrease in active tension.

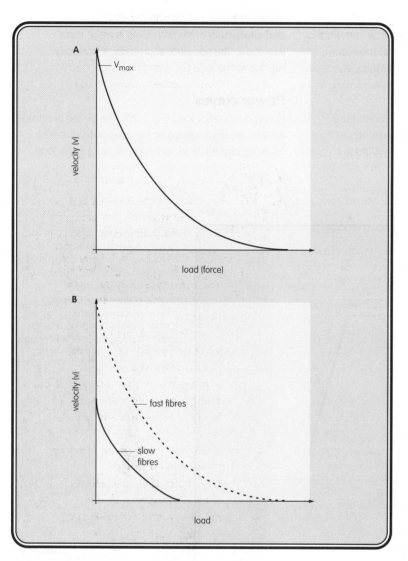

Fig. 2.31 Graphs showing that (A) speed of contraction decreases with increasing load, with maximum velocity occurring with zero load and (B) maximum speed of contraction in fast fibres is greater than that in slow fibres.

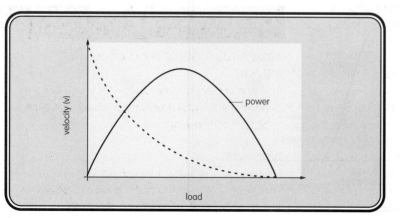

Fig. 2.32 Maximal power results from a balance between speed of shortening and load.

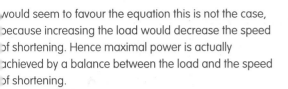

would seem to favour the equation this is not the case, because increasing the load would decrease the speed of shortening. Hence maximal power is actually achieved by a balance between the load and the speed of shortening.

Muscle plasticity

Muscle plasticity refers to changes in the characteristics of a muscle in order to match function. Factors that may be altered include muscle fibre diameter, length, strength, and vascular supply.

The fibre types may also be altered, but to a lesser extent as these are determined by the motor neuron by which they are innervated.

Fast fibres are interconvertible, i.e. fast glycolytic fibres may be converted to fast oxidative and vice versa. Slow and fast fibres are not interconvertible.

Effect of exercise

An increase in muscle mass occurs, owing to hypertrophy or hyperplasia.

Hypertrophy of muscle

Hypertrophy of muscle is an increase in the size of individual muscle fibres, resulting in an increase in the force of contraction. This is due to regular contraction of the muscle at maximal force.

Hyperplasia of muscle

Hyperplasia of muscle occurs to a lesser extent than hypertrophy. Hyperplasia involves an increase in the number of muscle cells. This is not due to mitosis but rather to a splitting lengthwise of large fibres.

Lack of exercise

A lack of exercise causes muscle atrophy. This is a decrease in muscle fibre size resulting from lack of stimulation.

Relationship of muscle characteristics to function

Sprinters have a greater number of fast fibres, as they require rapid contractions of large force, while marathon runners have a greater number of slow muscle fibres as they require sustained low-force contractions. The number of slow muscle fibres is largely genetically determined. By training, the effect of these muscle fibres may be enhanced by increasing their size and vascular supply.

Clinical relevance of muscle plasticity

Cardiomyoplasty involves the training of a skeletal muscle near to the heart, usually latissimus dorsi. The skeletal muscle can then be wrapped around the heart to replace diseased or congenitally missing myocardium.

- ○ **Explain the terms motor unit, innervation ratio, and size principle.**
- ○ **Discuss the different types of motor units and relate these to the different muscle fibre types.**
- ○ **Explain the effects of denervation and reinnervation on motor units.**
- ○ **Explain the terms isometric and isotonic contraction.**
- ○ **Describe how summation occurs.**
- ○ **What is the difference between tetanus and tetany?**
- ○ **Draw graphs to demonstrate length–tension and force–velocity relationships.**
- ○ **Define plasticity.**

CARDIAC MUSCLE

Structural organization of cardiac muscle

The heart consists of three layers—the inner layer (endocardium), middle layer (myocardium), and outer layer (pericardium) (Fig. 2.33).

Inner layer

The inner layer, or endocardium, is made up of endothelial cells which respond to pressure changes, stretch, and a variety of circulatory substances.

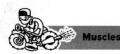

Middle layer

The middle layer, or myocardium, is thickest in the ventricles.

Outer layer

The outer layer, or pericardium, consists of the epicardium (visceral pericardium), which is intimately related to the myocardium, and the pericardium (parietal pericardium), which forms the outermost layer of the heart. The two layers are separated by the pericardial cavity.

Microstructure of cardiac muscle

Intercalated discs are low-resistance junctions between myocytes (Fig. 2.34). These allow rapid propagation of APs from cell to cell, hence the term 'cardiac syncytium'.

Types of cardiac myocytes

There are two types of cardiac myocytes—atrial and ventricular. The APs associated with these myocytes vary (Fig. 2.35).

Cellular physiology of cardiac muscle
Cardiac AP
Initiation

Under normal circumstances the AP is initiated in the sinoatrial node (SA node). APs occur at the greatest rate in the SA node; hence, it acts as the pacemaker, setting the rate in other myocytes.

Propagation

Propagation occurs rapidly, owing to the presence of gap junctions. The AP is propagated from the SA node to the atrioventricular node (AV node), before propagation to the bundle of His into the left and right bundle branches and Purkinje fibres to the ventricular myocytes.

Conduction is slow in the AV node, resulting in a delay of 0.1 seconds before excitation of the ventricles. This is important as it results in contraction of atria before the ventricles, thereby allowing greater emptying of the atria.

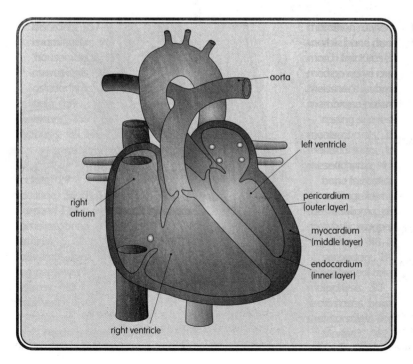

Fig. 2.33 Macroscopic organization of the heart.

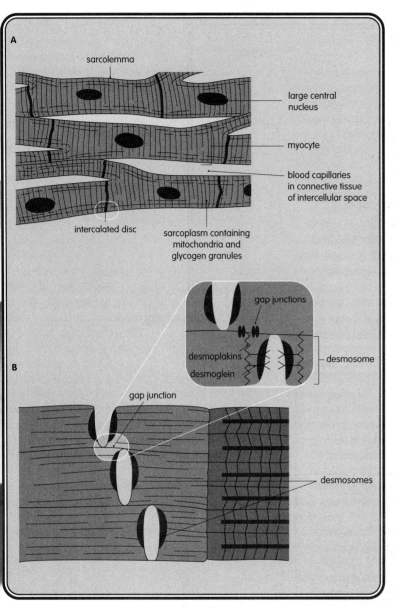

Fig. 2.34 (A) Microscopic structure of cardiac muscle. Note that there are far fewer mitochondria in cardiac muscle than in skeletal muscle. (B) Components of the intercalated disc.

Labels in figure A:
- sarcolemma
- large central nucleus
- myocyte
- blood capillaries in connective tissue of intercellular space
- intercalated disc
- sarcoplasm containing mitochondria and glycogen granules

Labels in figure B:
- gap junctions
- desmoplakins
- desmoglein
- desmosome
- gap junction
- desmosomes

Ionic basis

There are two types of AP in cardiac muscle.

AP in SA node and AV node: SA node and AV node cells have the property of automatic rhythmicity, owing to the leakiness of the membrane to Na⁺ in the absence of an AP and a decrease in K⁺ conductance. This results in a RMP that drifts from a threshold of −55 mV (lower than the RMP of ventricular and atrial myocytes) to −40 mV.

Ca^{2+} influx is responsible for the rising phase of the AP (Fig. 2.36).

AP in Purkinje cells and *atrial and ventricular myocytes:* Three types of channel are involved in the AP—fast Na⁺ channels, slow Ca^{2+}/Na⁺ channels (which are not found in skeletal muscle and are responsible for the plateau phase), and K⁺ channels (Fig. 2.37).

The AP in ventricular cells differs from Purkinje cells in

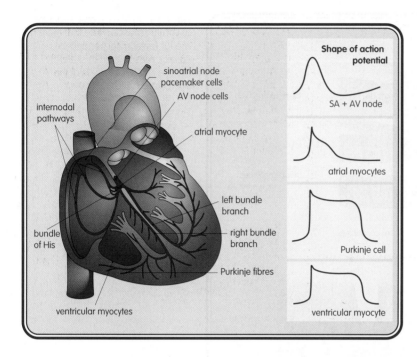

Fig. 2.35 Conducting system of the heart showing the location of the different types of myocytes and the action potentials associated with them. (AV, atrioventricular; SA, sinoatrial.)

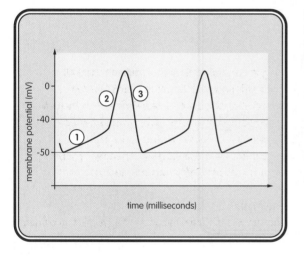

Fig. 2.36 Characteristics of the action potential seen in sinoatrial and atrioventricular node cells. (1) Drifting RMP due to slow Na^+ influx, or 'pacemaker potential'; (2) influx of Ca^{2+}; (3) repolarization due to K^+ efflux.

that the RMP is level in ventricular myocytes, whereas in Purkinje cells the RMP slowly rises to threshold, i.e. the cells are self-excitable.

Pacemaker tissue

Under normal conditions the SA node functions as the heart's pacemaker. In SA node pacemaker cells, APs are generated at a greater rate than in pacemaker tissue elsewhere in the heart. Hence the SA node sets the rhythm for the heart overall.

Pacemaker tissue is also found in the AV node, bundle of His, and Purkinje fibres. These are often referred to as latent pacemakers, as they can take over if the normal pacemaker fails.

Excitation–contraction coupling

Excitation–contraction coupling of cardiac muscle is essentially the same as skeletal muscle. This involves:
- Spread of the AP over the myocyte membrane.
- Influx of Ca^{2+}.

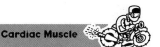

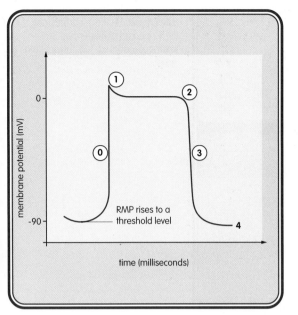

Fig. 2.37 Phases of the cardiac action potential in Purkinje cells. (0) depolarization due to rapid Na^+ influx; (1) initial rapid repolarization due to inactivation of Na^+ channels and a passive influx of Cl^-, (2) prolonged plateau phase with opening of slow Ca^{2+}/Na^+ channels. This prolongs depolarization due to Ca^{2+} influx and results in contraction of the myocyte. (3) late repolarization due to closure of Ca^{2+}–Na^+ channels and K^+ efflux due to opening of K^+ channels. (4) restoration of RMP. (RMP, resting membrane potential.)

- Contraction due to formation of cross bridges and sliding of filaments.

Bioenergetics of cardiac contraction

Cardiac muscle is mainly dependent on oxidative phosphorylation for contraction, as totally anaerobic conditions would not provide sufficient energy to sustain ventricular contraction.

Energy substrates vary according to dietary intake, e.g. during starvation, fat is the main substrate.

Cardiac muscle has a rich blood supply derived from the coronary arteries during diastole.

Cardiac muscle differs from skeletal muscle in that:
- The cardiac AP is 100 times longer.
- There is a long refractory period and therefore tetanus does not occur. However, upon increasing the frequency of APs there is an increase in intracellular Ca^{2+} levels. This results in an increase in the force of successive contractions and is known as the treppe or staircase effect.
- It is self-excitatory.
- The sarcoplasmic reticulum and T tubules are organized in dyads (at the Z lines), not in triads.

The sarcoplasmic reticulum is not as well developed and therefore stores less Ca^{2+}. Additionally, extracellular Ca^{2+} enters the cell directly through the T tubules via slow Ca^{2+} channels. Hence, the force of contraction in cardiac muscle is largely dependent on the extracellular Ca^{2+} concentration.

Inotropes

Inotropes are agents that increase the force of cardiac contraction (Fig. 2.38).

Mechanism of action: Inotropes increase the intracellular Ca^{2+} concentration. Digitalis glycosides, e.g. digoxin, inhibit the Na^+/K^+ ATPase pump. This results in an increase in intracellular Na^+ and therefore an increase in intracellular Ca^{2+} due to the action of the Ca^{2+}/Na^+ exchanger.

Sympathomimetics, e.g. dobutamine, act on β_1 receptors, which increase intracellular Ca^{2+} via a rise in cyclic adenosine-5-monophosphate C (cAMP).

Phosphodiesterase (PDE) inhibitors, e.g. milrinone, also increase cAMP.

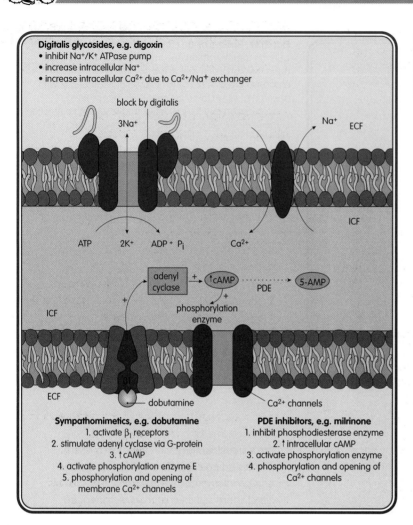

Digitalis glycosides, e.g. digoxin
- inhibit Na^+/K^+ ATPase pump
- increase intracellular Na^+
- increase intracellular Ca^{2+} due to Ca^{2+}/Na^+ exchanger

block by digitalis

$3Na^+$

Na^+ ECF

ECF

ICF

ATP $2K^+$ ADP + P_i Ca^{2+}

adenyl cyclase   +   ↑cAMP   ⋯⋯ 5-AMP
PDE

+

phosphorylation enzyme

ICF

ECF

dobutamine

Ca^{2+} channels

Sympathomimetics, e.g. dobutamine
1. activate β_1 receptors
2. stimulate adenyl cyclase via G-protein
3. ↑cAMP
4. activate phosphorylation enzyme E
5. phosphorylation and opening of membrane Ca^{2+} channels

PDE inhibitors, e.g. milrinone
1. inhibit phosphodiesterase enzyme
2. ↑ intracellular cAMP
3. activate phosphorylation enzyme
4. phosphorylation and opening of Ca^{2+} channels

Fig. 2.38 Inotropic drugs and their sites of action in the cardiac cell. (PDE, phosphodiesterase; ECF, extracellular fluid; ICF, intracellular fluid).

Function of cardiac muscle
Control of heart rate
Heart rate is affected by the autonomic nervous system.

Activation of the parasympathetic (vagal) nerves
Activation of the parasympathetic (vagal) nerves has the effect of decreasing heart rate, decreasing contractility, and slowing transmission of the cardiac impulse. These nerves mainly innervate the SA node and AV node.

Mechanism of action: Activation of the parasympathetic (vagal) nerves causes hyperpolarization of the myocytic membrane via muscarinic acetylcholine receptors. Anticholinergic drugs antagonize this effect.

Activation of the sympathetic system
Activation of the sympathetic system has the effect of increasing heart rate and force of contractility; β-adrenoceptor antagonists inhibit this effect.

Length–tension relationship in cardiac muscle
As with skeletal muscle, force of contraction increases with muscle fibre length (pp. 34, 35).

Starling's law
Starling's law states that the force of contraction is proportional to the initial length of the cardiac muscle fibre.

Muscle fibre length increases as the volume of blood in the heart chamber increases. Within physiological limits, the heart is able to pump out all the blood entering it.

Starling's law does not hold in situations where excessive stretching of cardiac muscle fibres is due to a decrease in actin–myosin interaction.

- ○ **Explain the term cardiac syncytium.**
- ○ **Describe the initiation and propagation of the cardiac AP.**
- ○ **Describe the ionic basis of the AP in the SAN to that in the Purkinje cells.**
- ○ **Describe the differences in contraction of cardiac muscle to that of skeletal muscle.**
- ○ **What is the treppe or staircase effect?**
- ○ **Explain the effect of the autonomic nervous system on heart rate.**

SMOOTH MUSCLE

The majority of smooth muscle found within the body is of the single-unit type (Fig. 2.39).

Organization of smooth muscle
Microstructure of smooth muscle
Smooth muscle cells are organized into small groups or bunches within the muscle (Fig. 2.40). These are surrounded by connective tissue containing the nerves and blood vessels.

The cells within a bunch are:
- Surrounded by an external lamina.
- Arranged in parallel to one another.
- Adherent at multiple sites.
- Able to communicate with each other via gap junctions (nexus junctions), which are present at sites where the external lamina is deficient.
- Able to contract together as a functional single unit.

Arrangement of smooth muscle in different tissues
Smooth muscle cells are arranged circumferentially in blood vessels and airways (see Fig. 2.40).

In the intestines and lower two-thirds of the oesophagus (the upper third comprises skeletal muscle), smooth muscle is arranged in two layers (Fig. 2.41). In the inner layer, cells are arranged

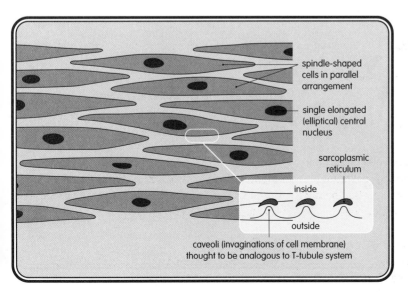

Fig. 2.39 Microstructure of single-unit (visceral) smooth muscle in longitudinal section.

spindle-shaped cells in parallel arrangement

single elongated (elliptical) central nucleus

sarcoplasmic reticulum

inside

outside

caveoli (invaginations of cell membrane) thought to be analogous to T-tubule system

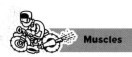

circumferentially and alter the diameter of the lumen, while, in the outer layer, cells are arranged longitudinally and influence the length. In this way both the diameter and length of the tract can be altered, causing movement of contents by peristalsis.

In the stomach, smooth muscle cells are arranged in three layers. These are the:
• Inner oblique layer.
• Middle circular layer.
• Outer longitudinal layer.

In the bladder, smooth muscle, cells are arranged in three layers. These are the:
• Inner longitudinal layer.
• Middle circular layer.
• Outer longitudinal layer.

Cellular physiology of smooth muscle
Initiation of contraction of smooth muscle may result from several mechanisms.

Autonomic nervous system stimulation
In smooth muscle, branching nerve fibres contain neurotransmitter within swellings called varicosities.

Released neurotransmitter diffuses to receptors on smooth muscle fibre, so there is usually no direct contact between nerve fibres and muscle cells (Fig. 2.42).

According to the type of receptor activated, the effect will be either excitatory or inhibitory.

The neurotransmitter released by a parasympathetic nerve may be ACh or, if released by a sympathetic nerve, noradrenaline. The two types of neurotransmitter have opposite effects in any one tissue.

If a section of smooth muscle has many layers, usually only the outer one is innervated. The resulting AP is conducted to other layers via gap junctions. In the intestinal tract, peristalsis is co-ordinated by the Auerbach's (myenteric) and Meissner's (submucosal) plexuses, which lie on either side of the inner circular layer of smooth muscle; closest to the epithelium.

Action of circulating hormones
The most common hormones influencing smooth muscle contraction are ACh, adrenaline, noradrenaline, angiotensin, and vasopressin; others include serotonin and histamine.

These act on receptors on the muscle fibre membrane, resulting in opening/closing of ion channels

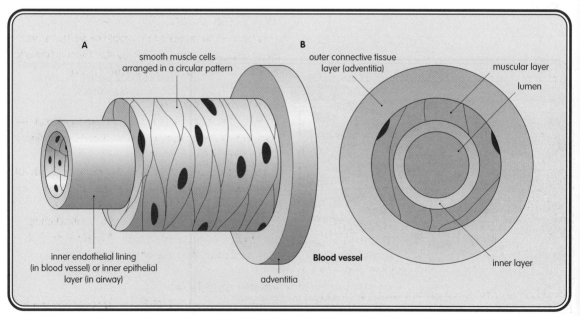

Fig. 2.40 Circumferential arrangement of smooth muscle cells, (A) longitudinally and (B) transversely.

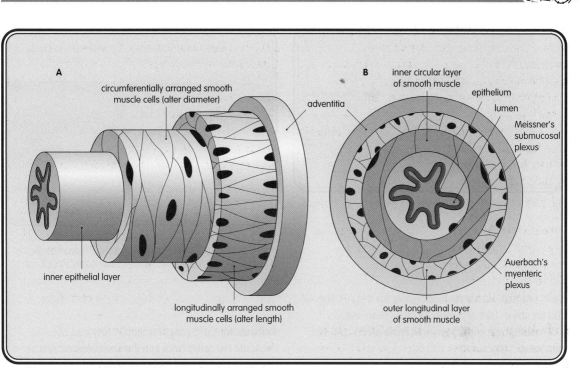

Fig. 2.41 Arrangement of smooth muscle cells in the intestine, (A) longitudinally and (B) transversely.

thereby initiating or inhibiting APs, and changes within the cell due to activation of second-messenger pathways, e.g. release of Ca^{2+} from the sarcoplasmic reticulum.

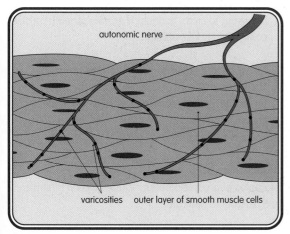

Fig. 2.42 Arrangement of autonomic nerve fibres in smooth muscle.

A hormone may have an excitatory effect in one tissue type yet an inhibitory effect in another. This depends on the receptor activated.

Local tissue factors
Local tissue factors involved in smooth muscle tone are carbon dioxide, H^+, and Ca^{2+} (Fig. 2.43). The mechanism by which these produce contraction is unclear.

Contractile apparatus
Smooth muscle has three types of contractile protein—actin, myosin, and desmin. Desmin is an intermediate filament (Fig. 2.44).

The proteins criss-cross the cell and are anchored at cytoskeletal points called focal densities or dense bodies (analogous to Z discs in skeletal muscle).

Focal densities transmit the force of contraction to surrounding smooth muscle cells. This allows smooth muscle cells to contract as one unit.

Smooth muscle AP
In smooth muscle, the RMP is usually about −50 mV to −60 mV (i.e. less negative than skeletal muscle), and

45

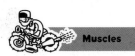

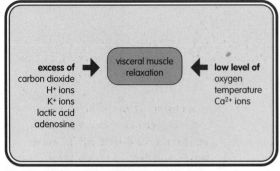

Fig. 2.43 Effect of local tissue factors on the tone of smooth muscle.

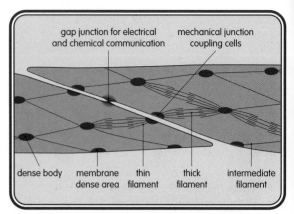

Fig. 2.44 Organization of contractile proteins in smooth muscle. (Adapted with permission from *Physiology 3e*, by R.M. Berne and M.N. Levy. Mosby Year Book, 1993.)

Ca^{2+}, not Na^+, is usually responsible for the AP. The AP can be spike- (skeletal muscle) or plateau-like.

Smooth muscle cells communicate electrically via gap (nexus) junctions.

Excitation–contraction coupling

During excitation–contraction coupling of smooth muscle, there is a rise in intracellular Ca^{2+}. Four Ca^{2+} bind to calmodulin protein present in the cytoplasm. This results in the formation of a myosin kinase–calmodulin–Ca^{2+} complex.

Myosin kinase phosphorylates a site on the myosin light chain. The phosphorylated myosin is then able to interact with actin to form cross bridges.

A decrease in myoplasmic Ca^{2+} concentration inactivates myosin kinase—the enzyme is only active when it is part of the calmodulin complex.

The dephosphorylation of myosin takes place by myosin phosphatase.

Regulation of intracellular Ca^{2+} concentration

In smooth muscle intracellular Ca^{2+} is elevated by:
- Mobilization of intracellular stores—Ca^{2+} is rapidly released from the sarcoplasmic reticulum upon activation of the cell.
- Voltage-activated Ca^{2+} channels in the sarcolemma.
- Receptor-activated Ca^{2+} channel in the sarcolemma.
- Caveolae—these are invaginations in the sarcolemma and are believed to be analogous to T tubules in skeletal muscle. The exact mechanism by which they control the entry of Ca^{2+} into the cell is unknown.

Intracellular Ca^{2+} concentration is restored by:
- Active pumping back into the sarcoplasmic reticulum.
- Active pumping of Ca^{2+} out of the cell.
- Na^+/Ca^{2+} exchange across the sarcolemma.

Smooth muscle contraction differs from skeletal muscle in that troponin is not a component of the thin filament and Ca^{2+} binds to the cytoplasmic protein calmodulin.

Disadvantages of smooth muscle contraction are that:
- Phosphorylation is a relatively slow process, therefore cross-bridge turnover and hence contraction velocities are low.
- ATP is required for both phosphorylation and powering of cross bridges. Therefore smooth muscle contraction is less efficient.

Advantages of slow cross-bridge turnover are that:
- The lower ATP consumption is adequately provided by oxidative phosphorylation hence no fatigue is shown.
- There is prolonged contraction.

Organic nitrates

Examples of organic nitrates include glyceryl trinitrate and isosorbide dinitrate.

Mechanism of action: Organic nitrates relax smooth muscle by increasing intracellular nitric oxide (NO) which interferes with contractile proteins and Ca^{2+} regulation.

Indications: Organic nitrates are drugs used in the treatment of angina and hypertension.

Adverse effects: There are no serious side effects from organic nitrates, although headache and postural hypotension may occur.

The organic nitrates act in the same way as the vasodilator NO produced by endothelial cells. Prostacyclin is also a vasodilator produced by endothelial cells. The vasoconstrictor released by endothelial cells is endothelin.

Functions of smooth muscle

The functions of smooth muscle depend on the site, such that:

- In blood vessels and airways it is important in maintaining tone and diameter.
- In the gastrointestinal tract it is important in mixing and propelling the contents along the tract via peristalsis.
- In the urinary system it is responsible for bladder emptying.

Myoepithelial cells

Myoepithelial cells are contractile cells found in mammary glands, sweat glands, salivary glands, and the iris. They are a layer of flat cells arranged around acini and ducts. The arrangement of contractile proteins is similar to that in smooth muscle.

Upon stimulation, myoepithelial cells contract and cause expulsion of glandular secretions.

Individual skeletal muscle fibres may be regarded as a syncytium as each fibre is made up of a number of myoblasts which have fused. However skeletal muscle fibres contract independently of each other and therefore skeletal muscle is not referred to as a syncytium.

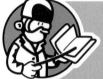

- Describe how smooth muscle cells are arranged.
- Illustrate the arrangement of myofilaments in smooth muscle.
- Describe the mechanisms involved in changing intracellular calcium levels.
- Describe how smooth muscle contraction differs from skeletal muscle and the effect of this.
- Outline the functions of smooth muscle in the body.

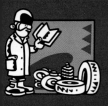

3. The Skeleton

The skeletal system is composed of various types of connective tissue, including bone and cartilage.

Bone and cartilage comprise cells embedded in an extracellular matrix. This matrix consists of an amorphous ground substance permeated by a system of collagen and elastic fibres. These fibres differ from general connective tissue because their matrices are solid, although they do share the same origin from embryonic cellular connective tissue, the mesenchyme.

Components of the skeleton

Bone
Bone is rigid and forms most of the skeleton. It is the main supporting tissue of the body and provides a framework for most of the body's tissues.

Cartilage
Cartilage is a resilient tissue and provides a semi-rigid support for certain parts of the skeleton, e.g. the costal cartilages, respiratory airways, and external ear.

Joints
Joints are composite structures that unite the bones of the skeleton. Depending on their form, joints allow for varying degrees of movement of the skeleton.

Ligaments and tendons
Ligaments and tendons are fibrous tissues that form part of the musculoskeletal system. Ligaments are flexible bands that connect bone or cartilage, stabilizing and strengthening joints. Tendons are the connections between muscles and their points of insertion into bones.

Functions of the skeleton
The skeleton provides:
- Support for the body, as it is a rigid framework.
- Protection for organs, e.g. the cranium over the brain and the thoracic cage over the heart and lungs.
- A mechanical basis for locomotion.
- Mineral storage—the majority of calcium, phosphorus, and magnesium salts are found in bone.

The development of blood cells, or haemopoiesis, occurs in the bone marrow. In the newborn, red bone marrow produces red blood cells, some lymphocytes, granulocytic white blood cells, and platelets. In adults, yellow bone marrow is mature bone marrow that has filled with adipocytes.

- **Name the tissues of the skeleton.**
- **List the functions of the skeleton.**

ORGANIZATION OF BONE AND CARTILAGE

Distribution of bone and cartilage
The human skeleton is bilaterally symmetrical. It comprises the axial and appendicular skeleton (Fig. 3.1).

The axial skeleton consists of the bones of the head (skull), neck (hyoid bone and cervical vertebrae), and trunk (ribs, sternum, thoracic and lumbar vertebrae, and sacrum).

The appendicular skeleton consists of the bones of the upper and lower limbs and includes those forming the pectoral and pelvic girdles.

With age, the proportion of bone and cartilage in the skeleton changes. In the fetus, most long bones are initially represented by cartilage that resembles the shape of adult bone. In the adult, the only remnants of hyaline cartilage are the articular cartilages of joints, the tracheal ring cartilages, and knee cartilages.

Cartilage
Cartilage microstructure
Cartilage consists of cells called chondroblasts and chondrocytes, which are laid in an extensive matrix. This matrix is composed of fibrous elements and a ground substance.

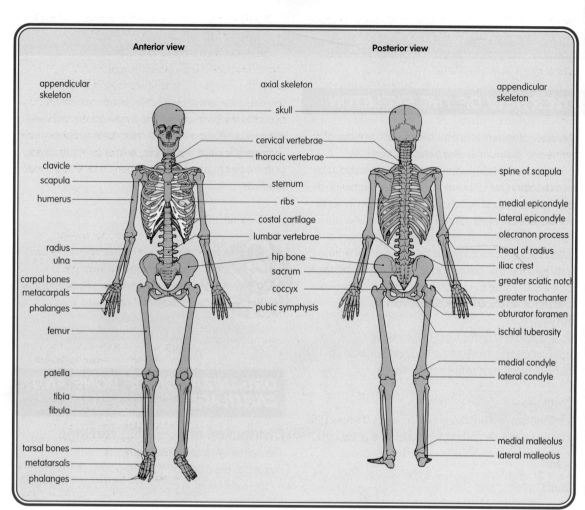

Anterior view   **Posterior view**

appendicular skeleton   axial skeleton   appendicular skeleton

skull

cervical vertebrae
thoracic vertebrae

clavicle
scapula
humerus

spine of scapula

sternum
ribs
costal cartilage
lumbar vertebrae

medial epicondyle
lateral epicondyle
olecranon process
head of radius

radius
ulna

hip bone
sacrum
coccyx

iliac crest
greater sciatic notch
greater trochanter
obturator foramen

carpal bones
metacarpals
phalanges

pubic symphysis

ischial tuberosity

femur

patella

medial condyle
lateral condyle

tibia
fibula

tarsal bones
metatarsals
phalanges

medial malleolus
lateral malleolus

Fig. 3.1 Anterior and posterior views of the adult axial and appendicular skeleton.

The chondroblasts and chondrocytes produce and maintain the matrix.

Cartilage formation and cell types

Cartilage derives from mesenchyme, embryonic cellular connective tissue. During development, the primitive mesenchymal cells become round, retract their extensions, and undergo rapid mitotic divisions. This process forms mesenchymal condensations.

Chondroblasts

Chondroblasts are the precursors of cartilage and arise from the differentiation of mesenchyme. They secrete cartilage matrix. The synthesis and deposition of this matrix separates the chondroblasts from each other and traps them within the matrix. Each chondroblast then undergoes up to eight further mitotic divisions to form groups of isogenous cells (i.e. developed from the same cell) surrounded by a smaller amount of condensed matrix.

Chondrocytes

Chondrocytes are mature cartilage cells occupying small cavities, or lacunae, within the matrix. Chondrocytes maintain the integrity of the matrix. Chondrocytes that are active have a basophilic cytoplasm (indicating protein synthesis), plenty of rough endoplasmic reticulum, and a large Golgi complex. Older, less active, cells are smaller and have a pale cytoplasm and reduced Golgi complex.

The sequence of differentiation and maturation of cartilage cells is most developed in the centre of growing cartilage. Towards the periphery of the cartilage, chondroblasts at earlier stages of maturation merge with the surrounding perichondrium (Fig. 3.2).

Perichondrial cells differentiate into chondroblasts, then chondrocytes, growing inwards from the periphery. Cartilage matrix, rich in collagen, lies between the cells. The lacunae are rich in glycosaminoglycans.

Matrix

Cartilage matrix is firm and solid, but pliable, causing it to be resilient. The matrix contains varying types and amounts of fibres and ground substance.

The fibres are made up of either collagen—type II (hyaline) and type I (fibrocartilage)—or elastin.

The ground substance is rich in glycosaminoglycans. Chondroitin and keratin sulphates are joined to a core protein to form a proteoglycan monomer. A hyaluronic acid molecule is associated with about 80 proteoglycan units; these are joined by link proteins to form a large hyaluronate proteoglycan aggregate. Cross-linking glycoproteins bind these aggregates to collagen fibrils in the tissue (Fig. 3.3).

Perichondrium

All hyaline cartilage, apart from articular cartilage, is covered by a layer of perichondrium. This is a dense connective tissue. Perichondrium is rich in type I collagen fibres. The outer layer contains fibroblasts and the inner layer chondroblasts.

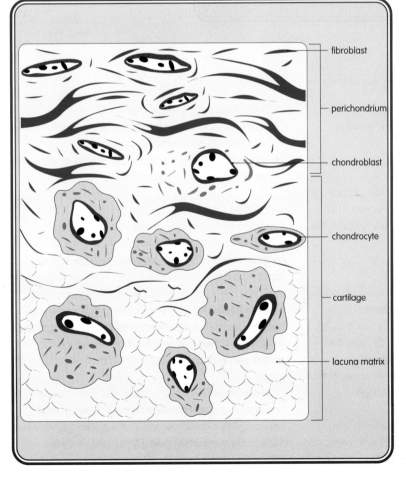

Fig. 3.2 Diagram of an area of perichondrium overlying hyaline cartilage. Perichondrial cells differentiate into chondroblasts, then chondrocytes, growing in from the periphery. Cartilage matrix lies between the cells; it is rich in collagen, apart from the lacunae which are rich in glycosaminoglycans. (Adapted with permission from *Basic Histology* 8th edn, by L.C. Junqueira, Appleton & Lange, 1995).

fibroblast

perichondrium

chondroblast

chondrocyte

cartilage

lacuna matrix

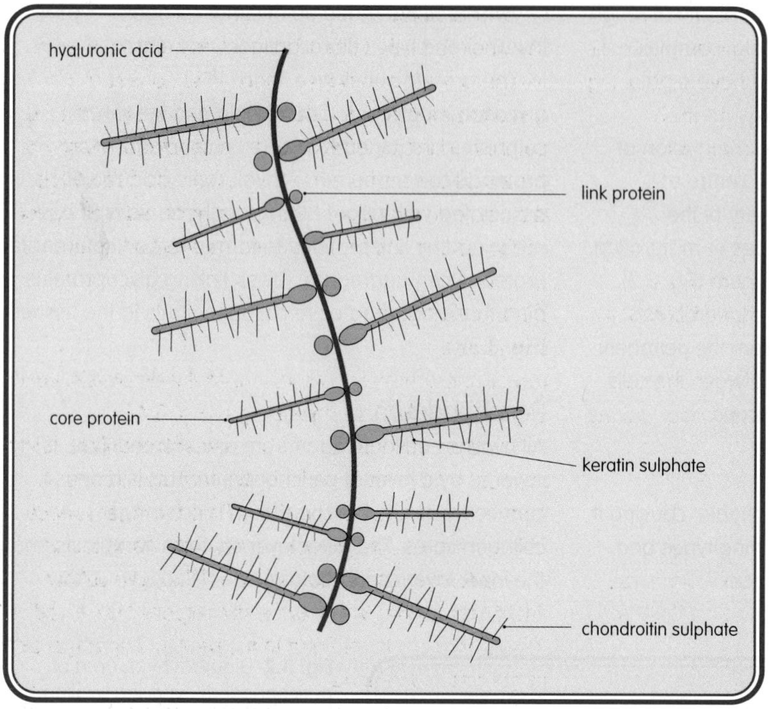

Fig. 3.3 Proteoglycan macromolecule.

Figure labels: hyaluronic acid, link protein, core protein, keratin sulphate, chondroitin sulphate

Growth
Cartilage can increase in size by either interstitial growth or appositional growth.

Interstitial growth
Interstitial growth takes place in the middle of cartilage by the mitotic division of mature chondrocytes. This occurs in relatively young cartilage, which is malleable enough to allow for internal expansion.

Appositional growth
Appositional growth occurs on the periphery of cartilage from the differentiation of perichondrial cells.

Blood supply
As mature cartilage is an avascular tissue, the exchange of metabolites between chondrocytes and surrounding tissue relies on diffusion through the matrix.

In sites where cartilage is particularly thick, e.g. intercostal cartilage, small blood vessels are carried into the centre of the tissue by cartilage canals.

Poor blood supply to cartilage:
- Limits the extent of its thickness, as the innermost cells need to be maintained.
- Makes repair after injury difficult. Injured areas are usually replaced by fibrous tissue.

Cartilage types
Cartilage type depends on the composition of its matrix components. Three types of cartilage occur: hyaline cartilage, elastic cartilage, and fibrocartilage.

Hyaline cartilage
Hyaline cartilage is the most common type of cartilage. It is characterized by a uniformly amorphous matrix and contains type II collagen fibres orientated along lines of stress.

Throughout childhood and adolescence, hyaline cartilage is present in the epiphyseal plates of long bones. It has a great resistance to wear and covers the surface of nearly all synovial joints, areas that are subjected to much stress.

Elastic cartilage

Elastic cartilage is composed of large numbers of elastic fibres and elastic lamellae embedded in matrix, making it flexible. It is found in the auricle of the ear, the external auditory meatus, the auditory tube, and the epiglottis.

Fibrocartilage

Fibrocartilage comprises a large number of type I collagen fibres embedded in a small amount of matrix. It is found in discs within joints, e.g. the temporomandibular, sternoclavicular, and knee joints, and also on the articular surfaces of the clavicle and the mandible.

Bone

Bone shape

Bone is defined according to its shape, i.e. long, short, flat, irregular, or sesamoid.

Long bone

Long bone is longer than its width; most bone in the appendicular skeleton is of this type. The ends of long bones are composed of cancellous (spongy) bone surrounded by a thin layer of compact bone. Their shafts contain a bony network along stress-bearing lines and surround cavities filled with bone marrow. The articular surfaces are covered by hyaline (articular) cartilage.

Short bone

Short bone has a similar-sized length and width, and is roughly cuboidal or round in shape. Such bones are found in the wrist and ankle. Short bone is composed of cancellous bone surrounded by a thin layer of compact bone and covered by periosteum. Hyaline cartilage covers the articulating surfaces.

Flat bone

Flat bone is usually thin, flat, and curved. It is found in the vault of the skull, ribs, sternum, and scapula. It consists of thin inner and outer layers of compact bone separated by a layer of cancellous bone called the diploë.

Irregular bone

Irregular bone does not fit into any of the previous groups. Vertebrae and sphenoid bone are examples of this type. Irregular bone is composed of cancellous bone with a covering of thin compact bone.

Sesamoid bone

Sesamoid bone is a small bone found in some tendons where they rub over bony surfaces. Tendons such as quadriceps femoris and flexor pollicis brevis contain the patella and the sesamoid bones, respectively. Most of a sesamoid bone is buried in the tendon; the free surface is covered with cartilage. Sesamoid bone reduces friction on the tendon and may also alter its direction of pull.

Bone anatomy

Long bone

Long bone comprises a shaft called the diaphysis; each end is expanded into an epiphysis (Fig. 3.4).

The diaphysis contains a large central medullary cavity surrounded by a thick-walled tube of compact bone. A small amount of cancellous bone lines the inner surface of the compact bone, forming a network of trabeculae.

In adults, the medullary cavity is filled with yellow (inactive) marrow, which is mostly adipose tissue; red (active) marrow is confined to the proximal epiphyses of larger adult long bone.

The epiphyses consist mainly of cancellous bone and have a thin outer shell of compact bone. Their articular surfaces are covered with a layer of hyaline cartilage.

In growing bone, the site of elongation of the bone is known as the epiphyseal cartilage (growth plate). When bone stops growing, the epiphyseal growth plate becomes ossified and forms the epiphyseal line.

The metaphysis, the flared epiphyseal end of the diaphyses, is very vascular.

Long bone is covered by periosteum and lined by endosteum.

Short, flat, and irregular bone

Short, flat, and irregular bone is composed of compact bone surrounding cancellous bone.

Bone microstructure

Bone is composed of cells called osteoblasts, osteocytes, and osteoclasts, which are embedded in an extracellular matrix.

Bone cells

Osteoblasts: Osteoblasts lie on the inner periosteum and the endosteum. They secrete an organic bone matrix in which they become entrapped, forming osteocytes. Active osteoblasts have a large Golgi complex, plenty of rough endoplasmic reticulum, and a basophilic cytoplasm. Resting (inactive) osteoblasts are smaller, flattened cells and have a paler cytoplasm.

Osteocytes: Osteocytes are found in small cavities called lacunae. Each cell has many processes, which run along canaliculi to connect with other cells via gap junctions. Osteocytes maintain the matrix, although they have less rough endoplasmic reticulum and a smaller Golgi complex than osteoblasts. When the cells die, the lacunae remain empty and there is resorption of the matrix.

Osteoclasts: Osteoclasts are large multinucleated cells with many branched processes. They are derived from the fusion of monocytes in blood and are therefore phagocytic. The cells resorb bone and are found in troughs, called Howship's lacunae, on surfaces where bone is being removed. Cells in the process of actively resorbing have a pale acidophilic cytoplasm, and many vacuoles and lysosomes for enzymatic digestion. They also have a ruffled border facing the bone matrix; an adjacent clear zone is responsible for adhesion to the matrix and provides a suitable environment of low pH for the lysosomal enzymes.

Bone matrix
Bone matrix has an organic component, responsible for flexible strength, and an inorganic component, responsible for rigidity and mechanical strength.

The organic matrix (osteoid) is composed of type I collagen embedded in a ground substance of proteoglycan aggregates. Also present are specific glycoproteins such as bone sialoprotein (rich in sialic acid) and osteocalcin (binds calcium).

The inorganic matrix is composed of deposited mineral salts, which make up more than half the weight of dried matrix. The most abundant minerals in the inorganic matrix are calcium and phosphate. These form hydroxyapatite crystals [$Ca_{10}(PO_4)_6(OH)_2$], the surface ions of which are hydrated to facilitate the exchange of water between the mineral crystals and body fluids. Bicarbonate, citrate, potassium, and sodium are also found but in smaller quantities.

Periosteum
Periosteum covers the outer surface of bone. Its outer layer contains blood vessels, nerves, and lymphatics, and its inner layer a few osteoblasts and osteoclasts.

Sharpey's fibres penetrate into the outer layer of bone to hold the periosteum, ligaments, and tendons in place.

The enthesis is the site of insertion of ligaments and tendons, and the articular capsule. Rheumatoid arthritis (enthesitis) commonly begins at the enthesis.

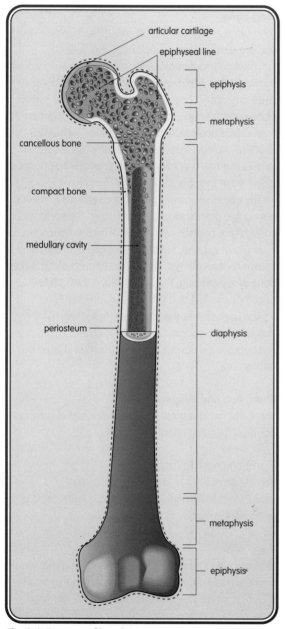

Fig. 3.4 Features of long bone.

Endosteum

Endosteum is a single layer of tissue containing osteoblasts and osteoclasts. It lines inner bone surfaces.

Blood supply and lymph drainage of bone

Several arteries supply blood to bone, which they enter from the periosteum (Fig. 3.5). These blood vessels include:

- The periosteal arteries, which enter the bone shaft at many points and supply the compact bone. At the midshaft of the bone, a nutrient artery passes through the compact bone to supply the cancellous bone and bone marrow.
- The metaphyseal and epiphyseal arteries, which supply the ends of the bone.

The arteries are accompanied by veins. They are

Fig. 3.5 Blood supply of bone.

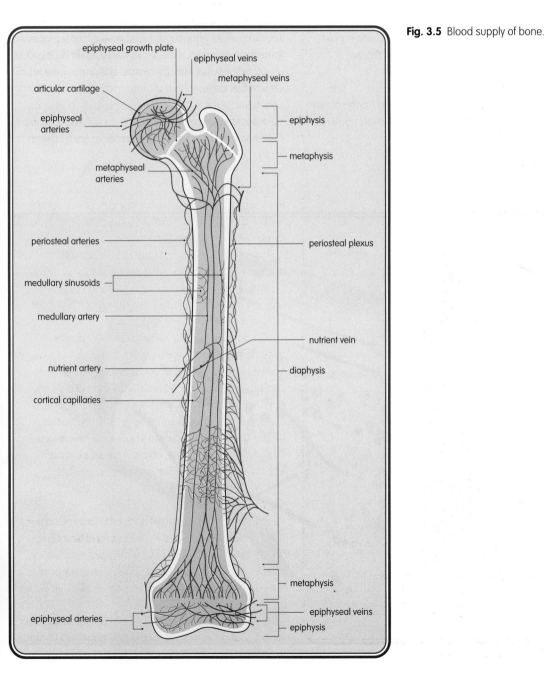

large and numerous in long bone and in areas of red bone marrow. The veins exit through vascular foramina near the articular ends of bones.

Lymph vessels are most abundant in the periosteum. They drain into the regional lymph nodes.

Nerve supply of bone

Many nerve fibres travel with the blood vessels to bone. They are mostly vasomotor, i.e. cause constriction or dilatation of blood vessels.

Periosteal nerves are sensory and contain pain fibres. They are sensitive to tearing or tension.

Classification of bone

There are two types of bone, depending on the pattern of collagen deposited—immature or woven bone and mature or lamellar bone.

Immature (woven) bone

In immature (woven) bone, an irregular array of coarse collagen fibres, a large number of osteocytes, and a low mineral content make it mechanically weak. Immature bone is the first type of bone to develop in the embryo and after fractures, and is gradually remodelled and replaced by lamellar bone.

Mature (lamellar) bone

In mature (lamellar) bone, collagen fibres appear in a regular parallel arrangement and have a highly organized infrastructure, which make it mechanically strong (Fig. 3.6).

Lamellar bone may be formed either as compact or cancellous bone.

Compact bone: Compact bone is composed of parallel columns along the long axis of a bone. Each column is

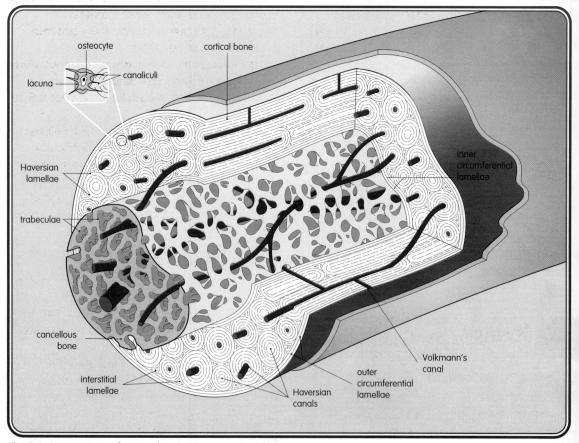

Fig. 3.6 Arrangement of mature bone.

made of concentric osteocyte layers fixed in the matrix in cavities called lacunae. The lacunae surround central neurovascular channels called Haversian canals. The units of lamellae and canals are known as Haversian systems or osteons. The vertical Haversian canals are linked with each other and with the endosteum and periosteum via transverse Volkmann's canals. Circumferential lamellae cover the outer surface of compact bone. Interstitial lamellae, which are remnants following bone remodelling, are also present.

Cancellous bone: Cancellous bone contains lamellae that form lattices called trabeculae. They are orientated along lines of stress and provide structural strength.

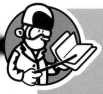

- Outline the distribution of bone and cartilage within the body.
- Describe the microstructure of cartilage.
- Give a simple classification of cartilage types.
- Describe the microstructure of bone.
- Explain the different types of bone and where they are found.

BONE FORMATION, GROWTH, AND REMODELLING

Types of ossification

Although all bones are derived from mesenchyme, the type of process they undergo for their formation, or ossification, can be either intramembranous or endochondral.

In intramembranous ossification, bone develops directly from primitive mesenchyme tissue, e.g. the skull bones and clavicle.

In endochondral ossification, bone develops indirectly from mesenchyme through an initial cartilage model, i.e. most bones.

The two processes result in an identical bone microstructure—both compact and cancellous bone can develop from either method.

After ossification, immature bone grows and is continuously remodelled by osteoclasts and osteoblasts until it is mature. This process continues throughout life.

The development of bone is controlled by hormones—growth hormone, thyroid hormones, and sex hormones.

Intramembranous ossification

Intramembranous ossification occurs within 'membranes' of condensed mesenchyme tissue. Ossification takes place from the centre outwards (Fig. 3.7).

Some mesenchymal cells differentiate into osteoblasts at primary ossification centres. Osteoblasts secrete new bone matrix, which calcifies and encapsulates the cells in lacunae. These cells then become known as osteocytes.

Osteoprogenitor cells beneath the periosteum divide mitotically to produce further osteoblasts, which lay down more bone. This process forms the outer surface of bone.

Islands of new bone tissue within the mesenchyme are known as spicules. Spicules are penetrated by blood vessels and haematopoietic precursor cells, which will become bone marrow.

As bone formation progresses, there is fusion of adjacent centres of ossification to form immature bone with a woven appearance.

Endochondral ossification

Endochondral ossification refers to new bone formation occurring from established cartilage. Chondroblasts develop in the primitive mesenchyme, (Fig. 3.8A) forming a hyaline cartilage and perichondrium model (Fig. 3.8B).

Osteoprogenitor cells and osteoblasts are formed at the midshaft of the diaphysis, creating periosteum and a collar of bone by intramembranous ossification. Calcium is deposited in the cartilage matrix (Fig. 3.8C).

Blood vessels grow from the periosteum and bone collar. They transport osteoprogenitor cells which

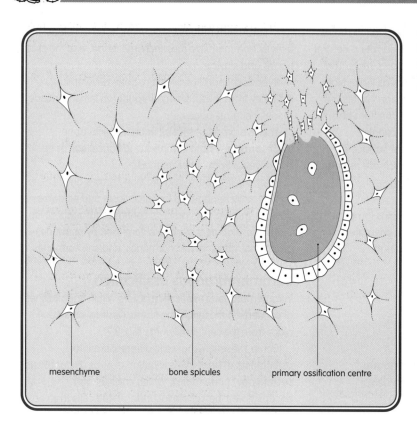

Fig. 3.7 Intramembranous ossification. (Adapted with permission from *Basic Histology* 8th edn, by L.C. Junqueira, Appleton & Lange, 1995.)

mesenchyme

bone spicules

primary ossification centre

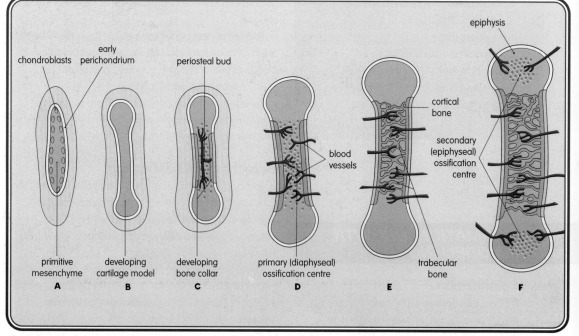

Fig. 3.8 Endochondral ossification. Parts A–F are explained in the text.

differentiate to create a primary ossification centre in the middle of the diaphysis (Fig. 3.8D).

Osteoblasts form lamellae on the calcified cartilage to make lamellar bone. This growth spreads from the centre outwards. The outer bone collar makes cortical bone. This happens prenatally, when the epiphyses are still made of cartilage (Fig. 3.8E).

Secondary ossification centres form in the epiphyses at different times after birth. There is endochondral growth until fusion of the epiphyses occurs at around 25 years of age (Fig. 3.8F).

Bone growth
Appositional growth
Appositional growth involves bone formation on the outer surface of bone. In long bone this results in an increase in width while in short, flat, and irregular bone, there is an increase in general size.

Endochondral growth
Endochondral growth involves interstitial growth of a cartilage model and then replacement with bone (Fig. 3.9). Overall this results in an increase in bone length.

At the epiphyseal plate, the diaphysis lengthens until the plate becomes fused, forming the epiphyseal line at puberty.

At articular cartilage, endochondral growth results in enlargement of the epiphyses.

Factors affecting growth
Factors that have an influence on bone growth include:

- Genetic influences, which determine bone shape and size.
- Dietary factors, such as vitamins D and C, which affect the formation of the organic and inorganic components of bone matrix.
- Hormones: growth hormone, thyroid hormones, and sex hormones usually stimulate bone growth, and also cause fusion of the epiphyseal plates to stop bone growth.

Bone remodelling
Immature woven bone undergoes progressive remodelling by osteoclastic resorption and osteoblastic deposition to form mature compact or

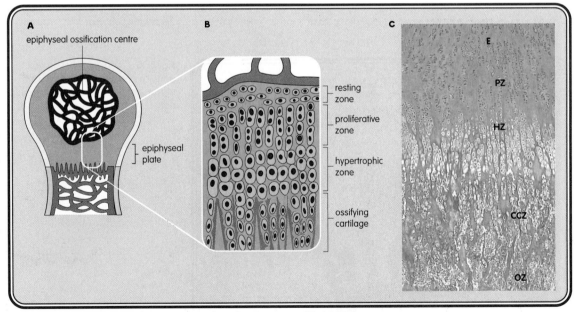

Fig. 3.9 Endochondral growth. (A) Epiphyseal ossification centre, (B) detail of epiphyseal plate, and (C) low-power electron micrograph. E, resting zone of the epiphyseal plate cartilage; PZ, proliferative zone; HZ, hypertrophic zone; CCZ, calcified cartilage zone; OZ, beginning of the ossification zone. (Courtesy of Dr A. Stevens and Prof. J. Lowe.)

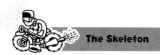
cancellous bone (Fig. 3.10).

Cancellous bone is laid along fibres of the mesenchyme, and compact bone is laid beneath the periosteum.

The primitive mesenchyme that remains in the network of developing bone differentiates into bone marrow.

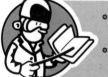

- **Name the two types of ossification.**
- **Describe the histogenesis of intramembranous ossification and endochondral ossification.**
- **List the factors that affect bone growth?**
- **Describe remodelling of immature bone.**

FUNCTIONS OF BONE

Maintenance of calcium levels

The skeleton contains 99% of the body's calcium. It maintains the levels of calcium in the blood within narrow limits so that muscle contraction and membrane potential activity can occur.

Normally, calcium levels in blood and tissues are stable and there is a continuous interchange of calcium between the blood and bone (Fig. 3.11).

When levels of calcium in the blood decrease, calcium is mobilized from bones. Conversely, excess levels of calcium in the blood can be removed and stored in bone.

One method for regulating blood calcium levels involves the transfer of calcium ions, firstly from hydroxyapatite crystals to interstitial fluid and then into blood. This takes place in cancellous bone and is a rapid mechanism helped by the large surface area of the hydroxyapatite crystals.

Other ways of regulating blood calcium levels are through parathyroid hormone and calcitonin release (Fig. 3.12). (Refer to *Crash Course: Endocrine and Reproductive Systems* for more details of hormones.)

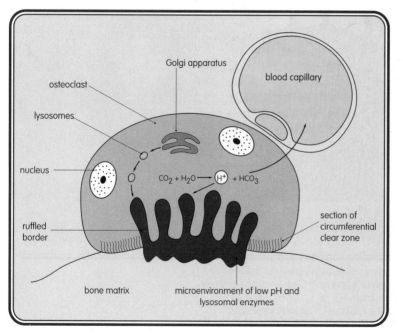

Fig. 3.10 Osteoclastic resorption in bone remodelling. (Adapted with permission from *Basic Histology* 8th edn, by L.C. Junqueira, Appleton & Lange, 1995.)

Golgi apparatus

blood capillary

osteoclast

lysosomes

nucleus

$CO_2 + H_2O \rightarrow H^+ + HCO_3$

section of circumferential clear zone

ruffled border

bone matrix

microenvironment of low pH and lysosomal enzymes

Parathyroid hormone

Parathyroid hormone (PTH) is the main regulator of calcium levels in blood. It is responsible for raising low blood calcium levels to normal. When blood calcium levels are high, less PTH is secreted.

PTH is a peptide made of 84 amino acids. It is secreted from the parathyroid glands in response to low blood calcium levels.

PTH stimulates osteoclast activity and results in bone resorption and calcium release into blood. It also increases renal reabsorption so that less calcium is lost in the urine. PTH also promotes the formation of vitamin D in the kidneys. Vitamin D increases the absorption of calcium from the small intestine.

Hyperparathyroidism, the excessive production of PTH, leads to demineralized bone and elevated blood calcium levels. The excess calcium deposits at other sites, such as arterial walls and kidney.

Calcitonin

Calcitonin is responsible for reducing high blood calcium levels to normal. It is a peptide made of 32 amino acids, and is secreted from the parafollicular cells of the thyroid gland in response to high blood calcium levels.

Calcitonin inhibits osteoclast activity and so opposes the action of PTH. It also decreases calcium and phosphate reabsorption in the kidney.

Excessive calcitonin production has no effect on calcium balance, so people with no calcitonin, e.g. thyroidectomy patients, do not need hormone replacement. The reasons for this are unknown.

Nutrition

During growth, bone is sensitive to nutritional factors. For bone and matrix formation to occur, the diet needs to contain proteins, calcium, and vitamins D and C.

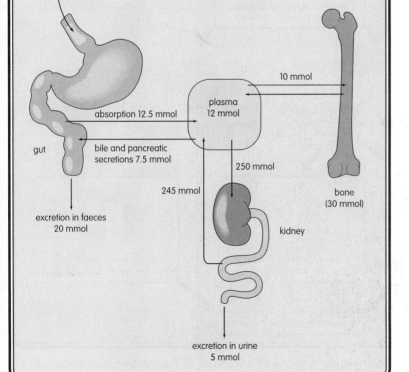

Fig. 3.11 Daily calcium exchange in the body tissues.

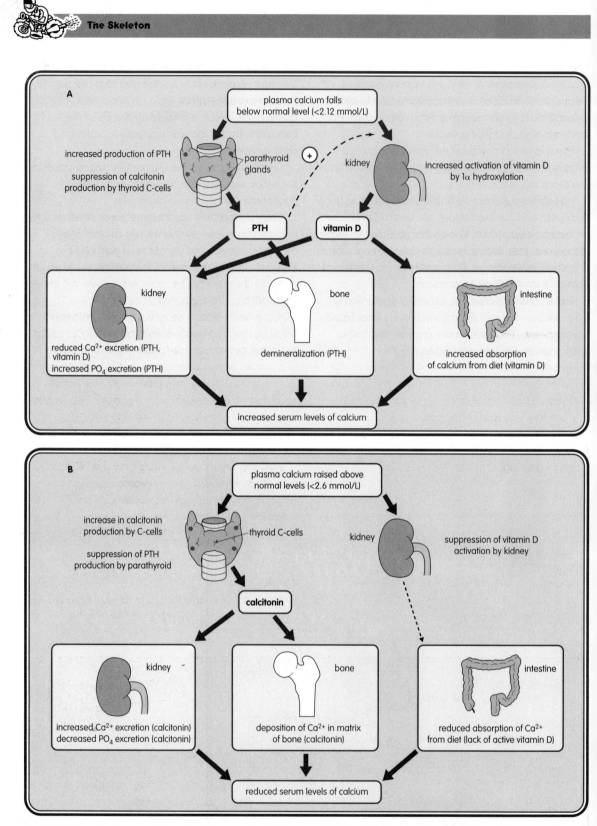

Fig. 3.12 Control of serum calcium levels by parathyroid hormone (PTH), calcitonin, and vitamin D where (A) serum calcium falls below normal levels and (B) where serum calcium rises above normal levels. (Adapted with permission from *Colour Atlas of Physiology*, by Depopoulous, Thieme, 1991.)

Vitamin D

Vitamin D is required for the absorption of calcium and phosphate from the small intestine and, to a lesser extent, kidney (see Fig. 3.12). It also stimulates calcium reabsorption from bone.

Small amounts of vitamin D occur in foods such as fish liver oil and egg yolks. Most vitamin D, however, is produced in the epidermis from 7-dehydrocholesterol, by a photolytic reaction mediated by ultraviolet light (Fig. 3.13).

Hydroxylation occurs in the endoplasmic reticulum of the hepatocytes of the liver to form 25-hydroxyvitamin D_3, which enters the circulation and is transported to the kidney by vitamin D-binding protein.

Further hydroxylation to 1,25-dihydroxyvitamin D_3 takes place in the mitochondria of the proximal tubules of the kidney. This most active form of vitamin D is called calcitriol. Its synthesis is promoted by PTH, and it has similar actions to PTH.

A decrease in vitamin D can lead to demineralization and poor calcification of bone. In adults this is called osteomalacia, while in children whose epiphyseal lines have yet to fuse it is known as rickets. Both conditions involve a loss of bone density, large epiphyses, and bowing of the legs.

Vitamin C

Vitamin C is essential for the synthesis of collagen in the bone matrix by osteoclasts and osteoblasts. It is a reducing agent, required for the hydroxylation of collagen residues, to allow calcification to occur.

Vitamin C is found in fresh fruit and vegetables.

A deficiency of vitamin C results in scurvy. The defective connective tissue leads to sore, spongy gums, loose teeth, fragile blood vessels, swollen joints, and anaemia. There is also interference with bone growth and slowed tissue repair.

Hormonal influences

Sex hormones

Sex hormones influence the time of the appearance of the ossification centres and stimulate closure of the epiphyses.

Sex hormones initially stimulate bone growth during puberty, when their production is increased. This accounts for the growth spurts seen at this time. However, they also stimulate closure of the epiphyseal plates so that growth stops. Oestrogens cause quicker ossification of the epiphyseal plates than does testosterone, which is why girls stop growing earlier than boys and are normally shorter than boys.

Precocious sexual development due to hormone-secreting tumours or administration of sex hormones tends to retard growth by causing early epiphyseal closure, whereas deficiencies of sex hormones caused by abnormal gonadal development tend to delay epiphyseal closure, prolonging the growth phase and resulting in tall stature.

Low oestrogen levels, common in immobilized patients and postmenopausal women, give rise to osteoporosis. In osteoporosis, although bone morphology is normal, there is a net decrease in bone mass caused by less bone formation and more bone resorption.

Growth hormone

Growth hormone increases general tissue growth. It is a peptide hormone released from the anterior

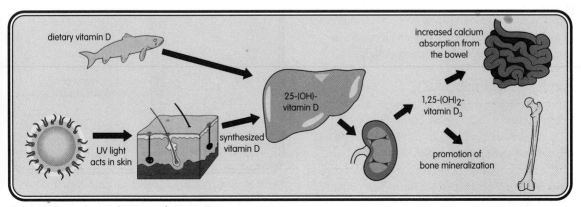

Fig. 3.13 Formation and actions of vitamin D.

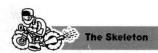

pituitary gland, and is regulated by growth hormone-releasing hormone and the inhibiting hormone, somatostatin.

Growth hormone stimulates interstitial cartilage growth and appositional bone growth.

During the growing years, too much growth hormone abnormally increases the length of long bone, resulting in gigantism. Adults with elevated growth hormone levels have acromegaly. In acromegaly, the epiphyseal plates have closed so the bones cannot grow in length and instead become wider.

A lack of growth hormone gives rise to pituitary dwarfism.

Thyroid hormones

Thyroid hormones regulate gene expression, metabolism, and the general development of all tissues.

Triiodothyronine (T_3) and tetraiodothyronine (T_4) are peptide hormones released by the follicular cells of the thyroid gland. They are regulated by thyroid-stimulating hormone (TSH), which is released from the anterior pituitary.

Thyroid hormone deficiency in neonates leads to cretinism and associated dwarfism.

Haemopoiesis in bone

Haemopoiesis is the formation of mature blood cells from precursors. In humans, haemopoiesis occurs in the medullary cavities of bone.

Red bone marrow is actively haematopoietic while yellow bone marrow, former red marrow, has become filled with adipocytes and therefore inactive. When stress is applied to the haematopoietic system, yellow bone marrow can revert to red marrow.

Although the number of active sites of blood production in bone marrow lessens from birth to maturity, all bone marrow retains some haematopoietic potential. Haematopoietic activity can reappear in anaemia and extramedullary haemopoiesis.

Location of haemopoiesis

In humans, haemopoiesis takes place in various sites according to the stage of development.

In the embryo, primitive blood cells arise in the yolk sac within 4 weeks of conception.

At 6 weeks' gestation, the embryonic liver becomes the major site of haemopoiesis. The spleen and lymph nodes also show some activity.

Bone marrow starts to produce blood cells when bones form medullary cavities after 20 weeks' gestation; it is the only site to do so by birth, when all marrow is red.

In children, the diaphyses of long bone, but not the epiphyses, show replacement of red marrow by yellow marrow.

In adults, haemopoiesis occurs only in some bones, e.g. the vertebrae, sternum, ribs, clavicles, hip bones, and upper femora, i.e. the axial skeleton (Fig. 3.14).

The bone marrow receives its blood supply from vessels that supply cancellous bone. Nutrient arteries enter the midshaft of bone through the periosteum and pass through compact bone to reach the medullary space.

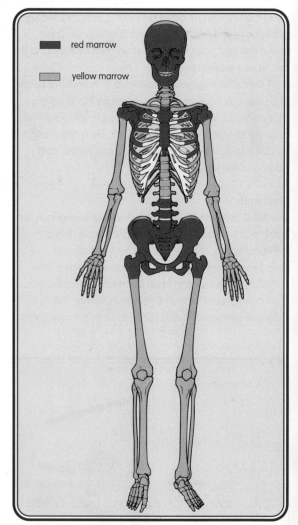

red marrow

yellow marrow

Fig. 3.14 Sites of haemopoiesis in an adult. (Adapted with permission from *Anatomy and Physiology 3e*, by R.R. Seeley and T.D. Stephens and P. Tate. Mosby Year Book, 1995.)

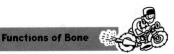

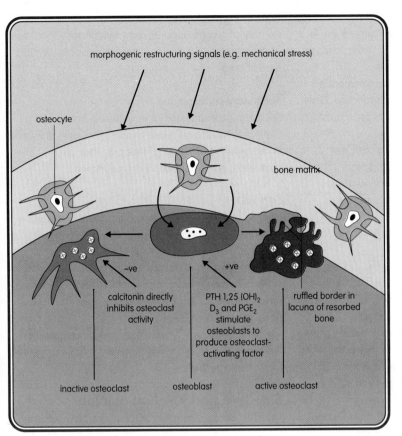

Fig. 3.15 Factors affecting bone remodelling in response to stress. [I,25(OH)$_2$D$_3$, 1,25-dihydroxyvitamin D$_3$; PGE$_2$, prostaglandin E$_2$; PTH, parathyroid hormone.] (Adapted with permission from *Essential Endocrinology*, by J. Laycock and P. Wise, Oxford University Press, 1996.)

morphogenic restructuring signals (e.g. mechanical stress)

osteocyte

bone matrix

–ve

+ve

calcitonin directly inhibits osteoclast activity

PTH 1,25 (OH)$_2$ D$_3$ and PGE$_2$ stimulate osteoblasts to produce osteoclast-activating factor

ruffled border in lacuna of resorbed bone

inactive osteoclast

osteoblast

active osteoclast

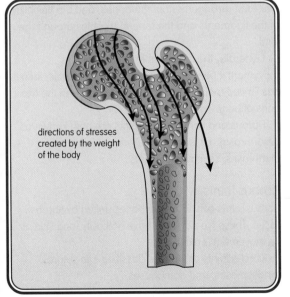

directions of stresses created by the weight of the body

Fig. 3.16 Orientation of trabeculae along lines of stress. (Adapted with permission from *Anatomy and Physiology 3e*, by R.R. Seeley, T.D. Stephens and P. Tate. Mosby Year Book, 1995.)

Response of bone to stress

Within limits, bone is a labile tissue that is capable of remodelling its internal structure according to different stresses (Fig. 3.15).

The two main mechanical stresses on bone are those from:

- The pull of skeletal muscles.
- The pull of gravity.

In response to mechanical stress, the increased deposition of mineral salts and production of collagen fibres make the bone stronger. In sites that are stressed frequently, bone is thicker, develops heavier prominences, and the trabeculae are rearranged (Fig. 3.16). Stress also increases the production of calcitonin, which inhibits bone resorption.

The bones of athletes, which are repeatedly subjected to high stresses, are notably thicker than those of non-athletes. Weightbearing activities, such as walking, help build and retain bone mass.

The removal of mechanical stress weakens bone through demineralization and collagen reduction. Bone is unable to remodel normally since resorption outstrips bone formation.

People who are bedridden or wear a cast, lose strength in their unstressed bones. Astronauts subjected to the weightlessness of space also lose bone mass. In these situations bone loss can be as much as 1% per week.

- ○ **Explain how calcium levels are maintained by PTH and calcitonin.**
- ○ **Explain the importance of nutritional factors during bone growth.**
- ○ **List hormonal influences on bone.**
- ○ **Locate and describe areas of haematopoiesis at different stages of life.**

JOINTS AND RELATED STRUCTURES

Classification of joints

Joints are the site at which two or more bones are united, regardless of whether there is movement between them. Joints are classified into fibrous, cartilaginous, or synovial, according to the type of tissue between the bones (Fig. 3.17–3.19).

Fibrous

Fibrous joints have fibrous tissue uniting the bones. This type of joint allows very little movement.

Cartilaginous

There are two types of cartilaginous joints—primary or secondary.

Primary cartilaginous

Primary cartilaginous joints unite two bones with a plate of hyaline cartilage. No movement is possible with this type of joint.

Secondary cartilaginous

Secondary cartilaginous joints unite two bones with a plate of fibrocartilage; there is also a thin layer of hyaline cartilage on the articular surfaces. A small amount of movement is possible with this type of joint.

Synovial

Synovial joints have a thin layer of hyaline cartilage on the articulating surfaces of the bones, which are separated by a joint cavity and covered by a joint capsule. The cells of the synovial membrane lining the capsule secrete a lubricating nutritive medium called synovial fluid. An extensive range of movement is possible with this type of joint.

There are several types of synovial joints, based on the shape of the articulating surfaces and the range of movements possible.

Structure and function of joints

The structure and function of joints are closely related. The range of movements available at a joint is related to its stability. This, in turn, depends on the shape, size, and arrangement of the bones, and the flexibility of the ligaments and the tone of muscles around the joint.

Generally, the more stable a joint, the less movement it permits. If a joint is solid (no cavity), then it has limited mobility. If a cavity exists between the two ends of bone, movement can occur.

Fibrous and cartilaginous joints are both known as synarthroses, i.e. solid joints. Synovial joints are diarthroses, i.e. cavitated joints.

Fibrous joints

Fibrous joints consist of two bones united by fibrous tissue. These type of joints have no cavity, and little or no movement is exhibited.

Fibrous joints are further classified into sutures, syndesmoses, and gomphoses.

Sutures

Sutures are interdigitating bones held together by dense fibrous connective tissue. This type of joint occurs in the

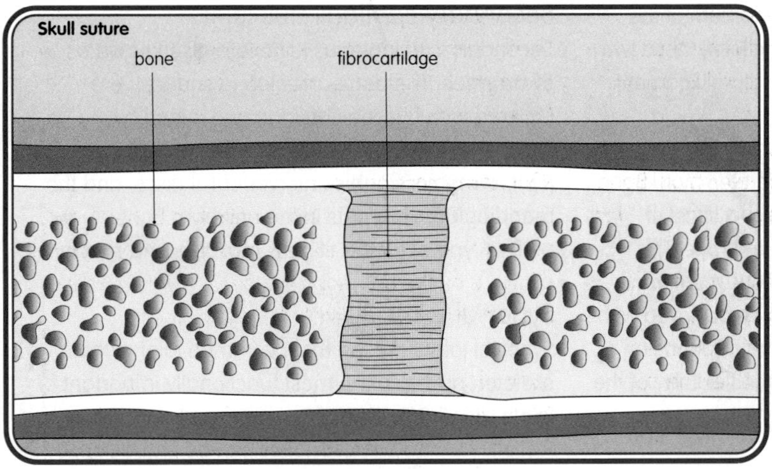

Fig. 3.17 Fibrous joint

Skull suture

bone   fibrocartilage

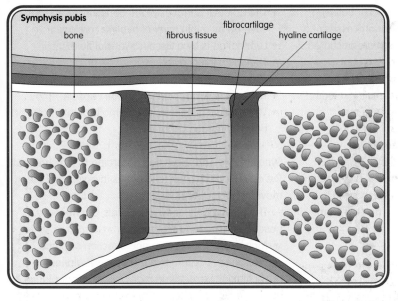

Fig. 3.18 Secondary cartilaginous joint.

Symphysis pubis

bone   fibrous tissue   fibrocartilage   hyaline cartilage

Fig. 3.19 Synovial joint.

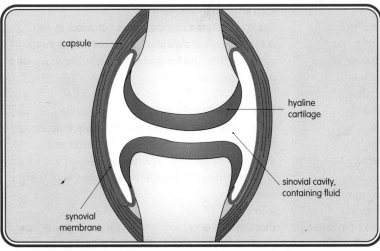

capsule

hyaline cartilage

sinovial cavity, containing fluid

synovial membrane

skull. The inner and outer layers of periosteum of the adjacent bones are continuous over the joint; these two layers and the fibrous tissue form the sutural ligament.

Syndesmoses

Syndesmoses are where bones are separated by a larger distance than in sutures, and are joined by a sheet of fibrous tissue—either a ligament or a membrane. This type of joint occurs in the radioulnar interosseous membrane.

A small amount of movement may be achieved with syndesmoses. The degree of movement depends on the distance between the bones and the flexibility of the fibrous ligaments.

Gomphoses

Gomphoses are specialized joints that occur between teeth and their sockets, and the alveolar processes of the maxillae and mandible. Gomphoses are anchored by the fibrous tissue of the periodontal ligament.

Movement of a gomphosis usually suggests a pathological condition, e.g. disease loosening a tooth.

Primary cartilaginous joints

Primary cartilaginous joints are also known as synchondroses. The bones are united by hyaline cartilage. They are found in the epiphyseal growth plate and costosternal joints. Synchondroses appear in the normal development of long bones, so most of them are temporary unions.

This type of joint is slightly movable.

In newborn infants, the sutures are called fontanelles. The bones within the sutures undergo intramembranous ossification, forming a synostosis. This happens in normal adults between the frontal bones. However, in old age there can be fusion between the coronal, sagittal, and lamboid sutures, and also in the sternum.

Secondary cartilaginous joints

Secondary cartilaginous joints are also known as symphyses. The bone articulating surfaces are covered with hyaline cartilage and joined by fibrocartilage. They are found in the manubriosternal joint, symphysis pubis, intervertebral discs, and the mandibular symphysis in the newborn.

This type of joint is slightly movable and strong.

Synovial joints

Synovial joints are the most common joint in the skeleton and also the most functionally important of joints (Fig. 3.20).

Fully formed synovial joints can be characterized by six features, namely:

- The articular surfaces of the bones involved are covered by a thin layer of hyaline cartilage.
- Lubrication is by a viscous synovial fluid.
- There is a joint cavity.
- The cavity is lined by synovial membrane.
- The joint is surrounded by a joint capsule.
- The capsule is reinforced externally or internally (or both) by fibrous ligaments.

Synovial joints are classified according to the shape of the articular surfaces of the bones involved and the movements that are possible.

The movements at synovial joints can be described as:

- Monoaxial, i.e. occur in one direction or plane.
- Biaxial, i.e. occur in two directions or planes.
- Multiaxial, i.e. occur in many directions or planes.

Plane joints

Plane joints are shaped like two flat surfaces (Fig. 3.21). They allow a sliding movement, i.e. monoaxial.

Plane joints are located in the sternoclavicular and acromioclavicular joints.

Hinge joints

Hinge joints have concave and convex shaped surfaces (see Fig. 3.21). They allow flexion and extension movements, i.e. monoaxial.

Hinge joints are located in the elbow, knee, and ankle.

Pivot joints

Pivot joints consist of a cylindrical projection inside a

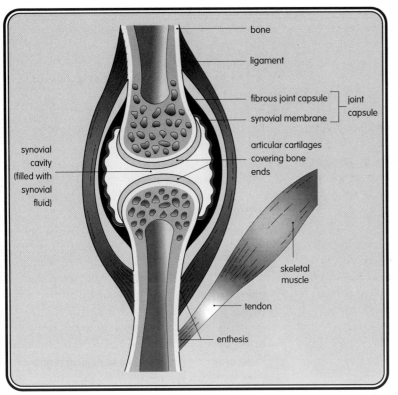

Fig. 3.20 Features of a synovial joint.

The labels in the figure are:
- bone
- ligament
- fibrous joint capsule ⎤ joint
- synovial membrane ⎦ capsule
- articular cartilages covering bone ends
- synovial cavity (filled with synovial fluid)
- skeletal muscle
- tendon
- enthesis

---

ring (see Fig. 3.21). They allow rotation movements, i.e. monoaxial.

Pivot joints are located in the atlanto-axial and superior radioulnar joints

Condyloid joints

Condyloid joints are shaped like two sets of concave and convex surfaces at right angles to each other (see Fig. 3.21). They allow flexion, extension, abduction, adduction, and a small amount of rotation, i.e. biaxial movements.

Condyloid joints are located in the metacarpophalangeal and metatarsophalangeal joints.

Ellipsoid joints

Ellipsoid joints have ellipsoid concave and convex surfaces (see Fig. 3.21). They allow flexion, extension, abduction, and adduction movements, but no rotation, i.e. biaxial.

Ellipsoid joints are located at the wrist.

Saddle joints

Saddle joints have concave and convex surfaces that are saddle shaped (see Fig. 3.21). They allow flexion, extension, abduction, adduction, and rotation movements, i.e. biaxial.

The carpometacarpal joint of the thumb is a saddle joint.

Ball and socket joints

Ball and socket joints are shaped like a ball sitting in a dip or socket (see Fig. 3.21). They allow flexion, extension, abduction, adduction, and medial and lateral rotation movements, i.e. multiaxial.

Ball and socket joints are located in the shoulder and hip.

Blood supply and lymph drainage of joints

The periarticular arterial plexuses supply blood to the joints. These branch into articular arteries. They pierce

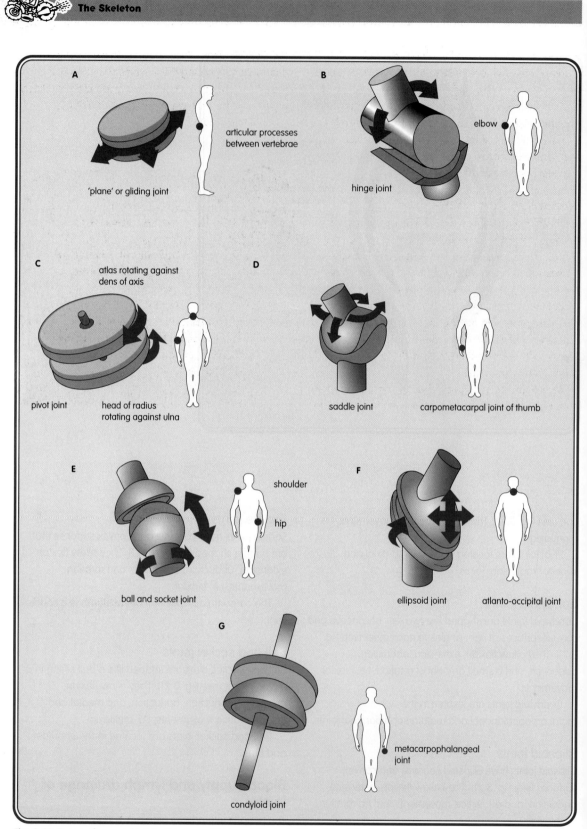

Fig. 3.21 Types of synovial joints: (A) plane; (B) hinge; (C) pivot; (D) saddle; (E) ball and socket; (F) ellipsoid; (G) condyloid.

the joint capsule to reach the synovium, and communicate with one another to create rich anastomoses around and inside the joint.

Articular veins accompany the arteries, so they too are present in the joint capsule and synovial membrane.

Lymphatic vessels are present in the synovial membrane and drain along the blood vessels to the regional deep lymph nodes.

Nerve supply of joints

Joints are richly supplied with articular nerves whose endings are located in both the fibrous capsule and synovial membrane. Articular nerves arise from the nerves supplying the overlying skin and the muscles that move a joint. This is known as Hilton's Law.

Both myelinated and non-myelinated nerve fibres are present in articular nerves. They have different endings that correspond to their roles in sensory input. The main types of input are proprioception and pain.

Myelinated nerves have Ruffini endings, lamellated corpuscles (rather like pacinian corpuscles), and some

like Golgi neurotendinous organs. These provide information regarding the movement and position of the joint relative to the body. Non-myelinated and finely myelinated nerves have free endings, which are thought to mediate pain.

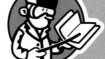

- Give a simple classification of all joints.
- Describe the different types of joints with examples.
- Describe the structure and function of synovial joints.
- Describe the blood and nerve supply and lymph drainage of joints.

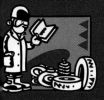

4. The Functioning Musculoskeletal System

Central control of movement

Motor control
Motor systems responsible for movement have three levels of control, which are organized both hierarchically and in parallel (Fig. 4.1), namely:

- The cerebral cortex.
- The brainstem.
- The spinal cord.

Cerebral cortex
Three areas of the cerebral cortex are involved in motor control—the primary motor area, premotor area, and supplementary motor area. The corticospinal tract originates from these areas and is the main descending tract involved in movement (Fig. 4.2).

Brainstem
The brainstem is the origin of other descending pathways, the extrapyramidal tracts, which play a role in posture, balance, and hand–eye coordination, i.e. vestibulospinal, reticulospinal, and tectospinal pathways.

Spinal cord
Spinal interneurons converge on spinal motor neurons, which innervate skeletal muscle. These interneurons act to inhibit certain muscle groups while activating others. In addition, movement can be modified by the basal ganglia and cerebellum.

Pyramidal tracts
Pyramidal tracts link the cerebral cortex, brainstem, and spinal cord. They originate from pyramid-shaped cells in the motor cortex, descend into the brainstem, where 80% of fibres cross to the opposite side, and then terminate in the grey matter of the anterior horn of the spinal cord.

Coordination of movement
The coordination of movement involves the cerebellum and basal ganglia.

Cerebellum
The cerebellum improves the accuracy of movement by comparing actual movement (via feedback from the spinal cord) with intended movement (via input from the motor cortex). This information is passed forward to the brainstem, so that movement is modified as it occurs.

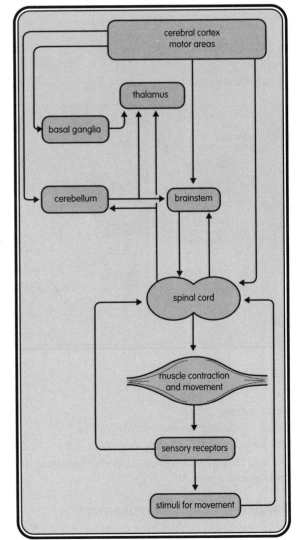

Fig. 4.1 Hierarchical organization of motor control in movement.

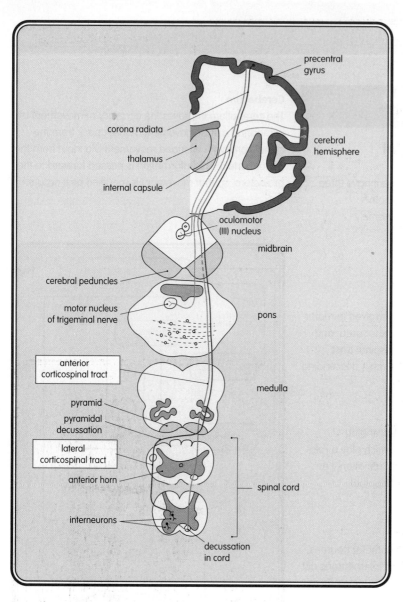

Fig. 4.2 Corticospinal tract.

The figure shows the following labels: precentral gyrus, corona radiata, thalamus, internal capsule, cerebral hemisphere, oculomotor (III) nucleus, midbrain, cerebral peduncles, motor nucleus of trigeminal nerve, pons, anterior corticospinal tract, medulla, pyramid, pyramidal decussation, lateral corticospinal tract, anterior horn, spinal cord, interneurons, decussation in cord.

Basal ganglia

Basal ganglia play an important role in the planning and coordination of movement and posture. They have connections with the thalamus and cerebral cortex.

Peripheral control of movement

Peripheral control enables the monitoring of movement, while it is occurring, via sensory receptors in skeletal muscle.

Types of receptors

Two types of receptors are found in skeletal muscle—muscle spindles and Golgi tendon organs. They are important in both proprioception and spinal reflexes. The reflexes of muscle spinde and Golgi tendon organs exert opposite effects (Fig. 4.3).

Muscle spindles

Muscle spindles are spindle-shaped organs made up of modified muscle fibres, termed intrafusal fibres (Fig. 4.4).

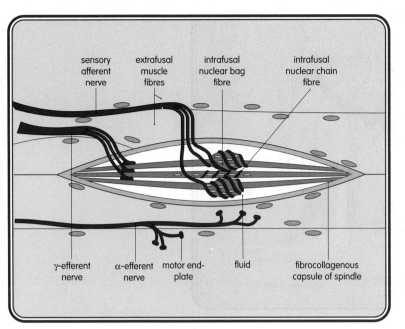

Fig. 4.3 Opposite effects of muscle spindle and Golgi tendon organ reflexes.

sensory afferent nerve

extrafusal muscle fibres

intrafusal nuclear bag fibre

intrafusal nuclear chain fibre

γ-efferent nerve

α-efferent nerve

motor end-plate

fluid

fibrocollagenous capsule of spindle

Intrafusal fibres are narrower than extrafusal fibres, and therefore do not contribute to muscle tension.

As muscle spindles lie parallel to muscle fibres they respond to changes in length.

Each spindle consists of several intrafusal fibres. These include:

- Two nuclear bag fibres, one for dynamic responses and the other for static responses.
- Five to six nuclear chain fibres for static responses.

Sensory innervation of muscle spindles is by group Ia afferent fibres, which supply both nuclear bag and nuclear chain fibres via primary endings. Group Ia afferent fibres show static and dynamic sensitivity, i.e. they respond to stretch and its rate.

One or more group II afferent fibres form secondary endings on nuclear chain fibres, although there may be occasional contact with a nuclear bag fibre. These fibres show static sensitivity only, i.e. they respond to change in muscle length.

Motor innervation of muscle spindles is important because it determines the sensitivity of muscle spindles to stretch (Fig. 4.5).

When the extrafusal fibres of muscle contract, the muscle spindle may no longer respond because its fibres are not being stretched. Activation of the γ-neurons causes shortening of

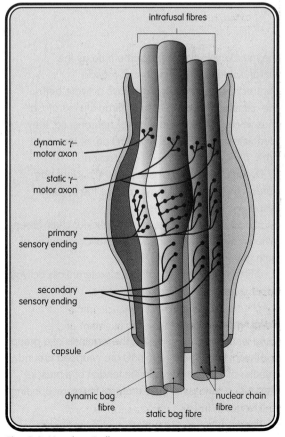

intrafusal fibres

dynamic γ– motor axon

static γ– motor axon

primary sensory ending

secondary sensory ending

capsule

dynamic bag fibre

static bag fibre

nuclear chain fibre

Fig. 4.4 Muscle spindle.

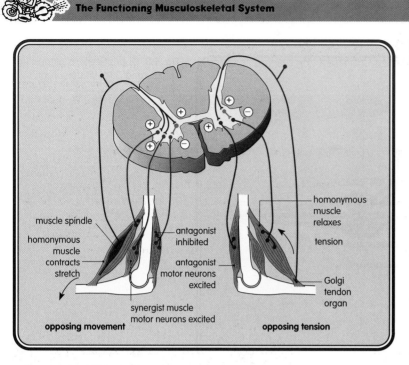

Fig. 4.5 Innervation of the muscle spindle.

the muscle spindles at the same time as the extrafusal fibres. During normal muscle contraction, descending pathways activate both the α-motor neurons, i.e. they stimulate extrafusal muscle contraction, and γ-motor neurons, i.e. they stimulate muscle spindle contraction, at the same time. This is known as α–γ coactivation.

Dynamic γ-motor axons supply the nuclear bag fibres. When activated, they enhance the dynamic response of group Ia fibres.

Static γ-motor axons supply the nuclear chain fibres. When activated, they enhance the static responses of both group Ia and II fibres.

Different descending pathways preferentially activate either dynamic or static motor neurons.

Golgi tendon organs

Golgi tendon organs consist of the terminals of a group Ib afferent fibre. These terminals are wrapped around bundles of collagen fibres in the tendon of a muscle. These lie in series with the extrafusal fibres, responding to changes in force.

There is no efferent innervation of Golgi tendon organs.

γ-Motor axons supply intrafusal muscle fibres while α-motor axons supply extrafusal, or 'regular', muscle fibres.

- Describe the hierarchical organization of the motor system.
- Locate the pyramidal tract.
- Describe the role of the cerebellum and the basal ganglia in coordination of movement.
- Describe the structure and innervation of muscle spindles.

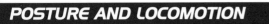

POSTURE AND LOCOMOTION

Posture
Control of posture
Posture is the relative position of the trunk, head, and limbs in space. To keep posture stable, the body's centre of gravity needs to be maintained in position over its support base.

Postural reflexes correct changes in posture caused by displacement of the centre of gravity—by either external forces or deliberate movement. Postural change is detected by musculoskeletal proprioceptors, the vestibular system, and the visual system.

Vestibular system
The vestibular system detects changes in head position, linear acceleration, and angular acceleration. The vestibular nuclei use this information, together with afferent nerves from the neck muscles and cervical vertebrae, to determine if the head is moving alone or if the head and the body are both moving. The nuclei can influence antigravity and axial musculature via a direct projection into the spinal cord.

Locomotion
Control of locomotion
Locomotion requires coordination between the systems controlling posture and those producing voluntary movement. This ensures that the body is supported against gravity and that the centre of gravity lies over the support base during propulsion.

A rhythm of muscle activity is needed, as each limb takes its turn in supporting the body and moving it forwards. The circuits that generate this pattern of activity are in the spinal cord and can be activated by higher centres, e.g. the brainstem. Sensory input is important in maintaining coordination of locomotion.

> Describe the role of the central pattern generator in movement.

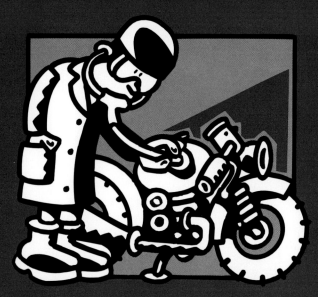

CLINICAL ASSESSMENT

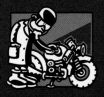

5. Taking a History

Things to remember when taking a history

First contact

When meeting a patient for the first time, you should:

- Always introduce yourself by name and status, e.g. medical student.
- Mention the consultant's name, as this reassures the patient you are genuine and provides a common link between you.
- Check that the patient is sitting/lying comfortably before you begin.
- Try to put the patient at ease by sitting a reasonable distance away, and take the interview at a relaxed pace; do not worry about any silences between your questions.
- Dress appropriately, as many patients feel uncomfortable giving personal details to young people—especially if they are scruffy and unshaven! Therefore you will obtain better histories if you are suitably dressed.

The patient's surroundings

Try to observe the patient walking into the consulting room, as any disabilities can be seen more easily during movement.

On the ward, look around the bedside for any clues to the patient's level of disability, or see what the patient brings to the consultation, e.g. an inhaler, oxygen, walking stick/frame, sputum pot, reading material, etc.

The patient's appearance and behaviour

Everyone subconsciously makes assumptions about people based on their appearance—you should try to be aware of someone's physical features and clothing.

Watch the patient's behaviour for clues while taking the history, e.g. is there agitation or distress, can you see any tremors, abnormal behaviour, or abnormal eye and body movements?

Structure of a history for muscles

Presenting complaint

When a patient presents with a muscular complaint, determine the symptoms experienced by the patient, e.g. muscle weakness.

History of presenting complaint

Nature of complaint

A patient with proximal weakness, i.e. weakness involving the upper parts of the arms and legs, will describe difficulties in:

- Getting out of the bath.
- Ascending stairs.
- Getting up out of chairs.

A patient with weakness of the hands may find it difficult to brush the hair.

Distal weakness in the limbs is suggested by:

- Difficulties in opening jars.
- Footdrop, in some cases.
- Tripping over rugs.

Patients with myotonia may present with an inability to let go upon shaking hands.

Onset of complaint

The onset of a muscular complaint will depend on the patient's lifestyle: e.g. athletes will notice a change in muscle strength at an early stage.

Onset is usually gradual in the muscular dystrophies, inflammatory myopathies, and myasthenia gravis. However, the inflammatory myopathies, periodic paralyses, and myasthenia gravis may also present suddenly.

The age of onset is also important: e.g. an underlying malignancy would have to be excluded in elderly patients presenting with myasthenic symptoms.

Pattern of symptoms

In the case of the inflammatory myopathies and muscular dystrophies, weakness is progressive as opposed to intermittent, as in the periodic paralyses.

Precipitating or relieving factors

Exercise: An important precipitating factor, particularly in the metabolic myopathies, periodic paralyses, and myasthenia gravis, is exercise. The symptoms of Lambert–Eaton myasthenic syndrome improve with exercise.

Temperature: The myotonia associated with Thomsen's disease and paramyotonia congenita is worse in the cold.

Other associated symptoms

Muscle pain may be a feature of the metabolic myopathies, viral myalgias, and alcohol excess myopathy. Dysphagia, dysarthria, and respiratory symptoms may be present, depending on the muscle groups involved.

Bone pain would suggest osteomalacia-induced myopathy.

Past medical history

A history of HIV infection should be excluded, as the infection itself, or its treatment, e.g. zidovudine, may be responsible for myopathy.

Drug history

A range of drugs, e.g. steroids, cholesterol-lowering agents, chloroquine, and lithium, can result in proximal myopathy.

Family history

If other family members are affected by a muscular disorder, a family tree should be constructed. The sex of the patient and affected relatives should be noted.

Social history

Alcohol: When ascertaining the patient's social history, you should ask about alcohol consumption. How many units does the patient consume and how often?

Sexual practices: You should try to establish if the patient is at risk of infection with HIV.

Exercise: Ask the patient about exercise, as this can help exclude disuse atrophy.

Systems review

You should try to establish whether the patient has symptoms of other connective tissue disorders: e.g. dark urine is suggestive of myoglobinuria and is associated with metabolic myopathies and acute alcoholic myopathy.

Does the patient have symptoms of endocrine disease, e.g. Cushing's syndrome or thyroid abnormalities?

Summary of patient's history

Always write a summary of a patient's history when presenting the case.

Structure of a history for joints
Presenting complaint

Presenting complaints of joint disorders are usually:
- Pain.
- Swelling.
- Stiffness.
- Deformity.
- Loss of function.
- Numbness or paraesthesia.

For each of these, ask when and where the symptom started, if anything makes it better or worse, and how daily life is affected.

History of presenting complaint
Past medical history

Enquire about any previous injuries, as some may predispose to new disorders.

Family history

Genetic disorders should be considered in joint complaints.

Social history

Information about a patient's social life, e.g. occupation and hobbies, can help to assist in a diagnosis.

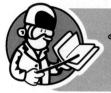

○ **Name the main points for a good history taking.**

COMMON PRESENTING COMPLAINTS

Monoarticular arthritis

Monoarticular arthritis is a common presenting joint complaint (Fig. 5.1). It can be classified into acute and chronic forms.

Acute monoarticular arthritis

Ninety per cent of cases of acute monoarticular arthritis are due to one of several causes. These include:

- Sepsis, e.g. from staphylococcal infection.
- Crystal-induced, e.g. gout.
- Trauma.

Chronic monoarticular arthritis

If monoarticular arthritis occurs for more than 2 months, it is referred to as chronic (Figs 5.2, 5.3). The causes of chronic monoarticular arthritis include those of both acute monoarticular arthritis and polyarticular arthritis.

Polyarticular arthritis

Polyarticular arthritis is inflammation of more than one joint. It can be classified into an acute or chronic form: when the condition lasts for more than 6–8 weeks, it is described as chronic.

Causes of acute polyarthritis include rheumatoid arthritis, the spondylarthritides, viral arthritis (e.g. rubella and hepatitis B), systemic lupus erythematosus, and acute rheumatic fever.

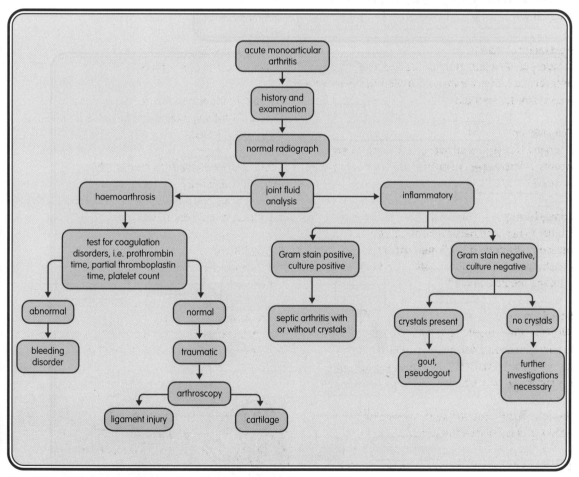

Fig. 5.1 Stages involved in determining a diagnosis of monoarticular arthritis.

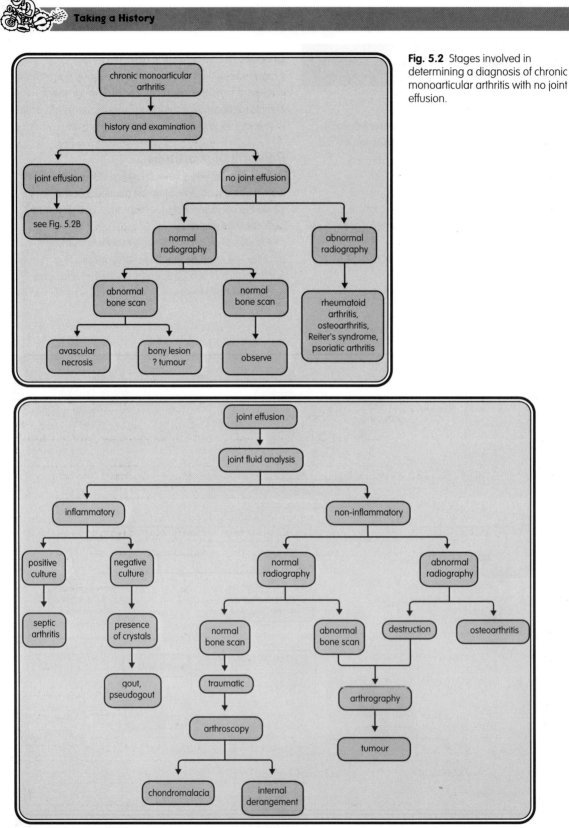

Fig. 5.2 Stages involved in determining a diagnosis of chronic monoarticular arthritis with no joint effusion.

Fig. 5.3 Stages involved in determining a diagnosis of chronic monoarticular arthritis with an associated joint effusion

Causes of chronic polyarthritis include osteoarthritis, rheumatoid arthritis, some of the spondylarthritides (e.g. psoriatic arthritis, Reiter's syndrome), sarcoid arthritis, and systemic lupus erythematosus.

The diagnosis of polyarticular arthritis is aided by a thorough history, as this type of arthritis is often associated with extra-articular features that would indicate the most likely cause (Fig. 5.4).

Muscle weakness

Patients with muscle weakness can be divided into two categories: those with 'true' muscle weakness and those with normal muscle strength.

Muscle weakness may result from disorders occurring anywhere along the motor cortex, corticospinal tracts, anterior horn cells, peripheral nerves, neuromuscular junction, and muscle. (Only the last two of these sites will be considered here.)

Diagnosis of muscle weakness is aided by considering the distribution of the weakness (Fig. 5.5).

Further investigations, involving electromyography and muscle biopsy, are required for the definitive diagnosis of muscular weakness.

Systemic symptoms that may aid diagnosis of polyarthritis		
System	**Symptoms**	**Possible diagnoses**
general	unexplained weight loss, fatiguability	systemic lupus erythematosus (SLE), rheumatoid arthritis, ankylosing spondylitis, Reiter's syndrome, sarcoidosis
eyes	dryness	Sjögren's syndrome
	pain	SLE, rheumatoid arthritis, ankylosing spondylitis, Reiter's syndrome, Behçet 's syndrome, sarcoidosis
mucocutaneous	dry mouth	Sjögren's syndrome
	rash	SLE, dermatomyositis, psoriasis, Reiter's syndrome, Sjögren's syndrome
	nail pitting	psoriasis, Reiter's syndrome
	subcutaneous nodules	rheumatoid arthritis, SLE, gout, sarcoidosis
respiratory	shortness of breath, pleuritic pain	SLE, rheumatoid arthritis
gastrointestinal	symptoms of inflammatory bowel disease	enteropathic arthritis
genitourinary	dysuria	Reiter's syndrome
	painful intercourse	Sjögren's syndrome, Behçet's syndrome
musculoskeletal	muscle weakness	polymyositis, dermatomyositis, rheumatoid arthritis, SLE, sarcoidosis
	muscle tenderness, stiffness	rheumatoid arthritis, SLE
	joint symptoms	inflammatory arthritis
nervous	headaches and visual problems	SLE

Fig. 5.4 Systemic symptoms that may aid in a diagnosis of polyarthritis.

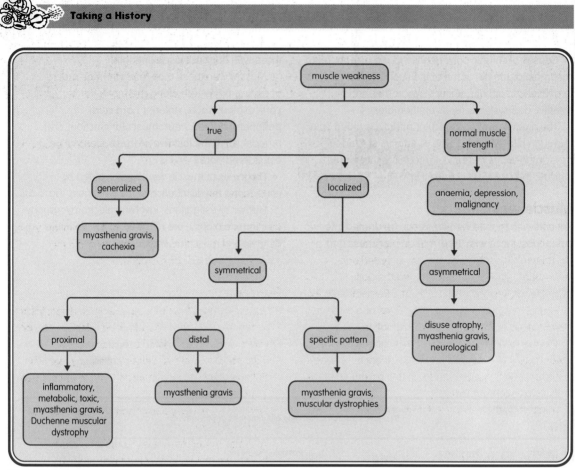

Fig. 5.5 Stages involved in determining a diagnosis of muscle weakness.

° **What are the stages involved in making the diagnosis of monoarticular arthritis?**

° **What are the systemic symptoms associated with polyarthritis?**

° **Which features of the history may aid in the diagnosis of muscle weakness?**

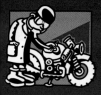

6. Examination of the Patient

GENERAL EXAMINATION OF JOINTS AND THE MUSCULOSKELETAL SYSTEM

Clinical examination

It is useful to approach the clinical examination of a patient in a systematic way so that important signs are not missed. All findings should be recorded and summarized. You should make sure the patient feels at ease and explain instructions clearly. Remember to look at the patient's face when eliciting signs and explain your findings at the end of the examination.

When examining limbs, start with either the upper or lower limb, and examine both limbs at once. It is easier to find an abnormality when there is a normal structure available for comparison.

Joints should be examined from the front, back, and sides.

General examination of joints

The routine for examination of joints involves:
- Inspection.
- Palpation.
- Movement.
- Stressing.

This routine is usually followed by X-rays. It is advisable to examine painful areas last.

Inspection

The area for examination should be adequately exposed and viewed in good light. Note should be made of:
- The alignment of the bones—look for any deformities and shortening. Subluxation is present when displaced parts of the joint surfaces remain partially in contact.
- The position of the joint and limbs at rest—is there any unusual posture?
- The joint contour to check for swellings and abnormalities—are there any effusions and general or localized swellings?
- Scars or sinuses—are these from operations (linear

scar), injury (irregular scar), or suppurations (broad, adherent, puckered scar)?
- The skin.
- Muscle wasting.

The terms valgus and varus refer to the deviation of the limb distal to a joint—away from or towards the midline, respectively (see Chapter 2).

Palpation

Palpation includes both measurements and sensibility.

Preferably with warm hands, initially feel gently and then more firmly. You should consider:
- Skin temperature changes by noting any warmth (inflammation, rapidly growing tumour) or coldness in local areas.
- Swellings—are they bony abnormalities or diffuse joint swellings?
- Areas of tenderness—these should be precisely located so as to relate them to anatomical structures.
- Pain—check the patient's face for apprehension.

Measurements

Measurements of limb length and width are carried out when there are discrepancies between both sides. Length is especially important in the lower limbs, and width provides information on muscle wasting, soft tissue swellings, or bone thickenings. Refer to fixed points when measuring and check that the findings are reproducible.

Sensibility

An area's sensibility to light touch and to pinpricks should be assessed. You should precisely locate areas of blunting or loss of sensation.

Movement

Both active and passive ranges of movement must be recorded for the directional planes of each joint. These should be equal: passive movement exceeds active when there is muscle paralysis, or torn or slack tendons.

A goniometer, a hinged rod with a protractor in the centre, is the instrument used for measuring the range of joint movements. Measurements usually begin from the joint positioned in extension, and movement is expressed as degrees of flexion from this point.

The normal ranges of joint movements need to be fully understood, and both sides tested. Restricted movements in all directions are suggestive of arthritis, while restrictive movements in some directions and free movements in others suggest a mechanical disorder.

Pain and crepitations must also be noted. Joint crepitations are coarse and diffuse while those of the tendons are fine and located to the tendon sheath.

Straining and strength

Straining of the ligaments provides information about joint stability. When assessing ligaments, the muscles moving the joint must be relaxed as contracted ones can conceal unstable ligaments.

Pain is usually present in ligaments that are recently injured, while those that are torn or stretched produce an increased range of movements.

The strength of muscle can be tested by asking the patient to move a joint against the resistance of the examiner. Muscle weakness is easily detectable and a very important sign of motor impairment.

Muscle power is graded according to the Medical Research Council as:

- 0, no power.
- 1, a flicker of contraction.
- 2, slight power to move a joint with gravity eliminated—this is when the joint is supported, usually by the edge of a bed or manually by the observer.
- 3, sufficient power to move a joint against gravity.
- 4, power to move a joint against gravity plus added resistance.
- 5, normal muscle power.

X-rays

Anteroposterior and lateral views of a joint are routinely taken during an X-ray examination, except for the hands and feet. Bones, joints, and soft tissues are also examined.

Bones

It is important to observe the general outline of bones—are there areas of increased or decreased density?

Joints

When assessing joints you should check for:

- Narrowing of the joint space, indicating loss of cartilage thickness.
- Joint margin erosion, typical of rheumatoid arthritis.
- New bone-forming osteophytes, typical of osteoarthritis.
- Flattening or thickening of bone.
- Bone erosion or cavitation.

Soft tissues

In the soft tissues, areas of calcification, foreign bodies, and increased density (suggestive of fluid), should all be noted.

- Explain why an adaptable routine should be used when examining joints.
- Describe the salient signs elicited after inspection, palpution, movement and stressing.

REGIONAL EXAMINATION OF JOINTS AND THE MUSCULOSKELETAL SYSTEM

The principles of general examination are applied to local areas. This section focuses on specific features that should be noted and manoeuvres that should be performed.

Examination of the back

Cervical spine

Inspection

During inspection of the cervical spine you should note any deformities such as torticollis, a 'cock-robin' posture (lateral flexion due to cervical erosion from rheumatoid arthritis), and hyperextension (compensation for a small thorax in ankylosing spondylitis).

Palpation

During palpation of the cervical spine you should check for midline tenderness from a sprain or whiplash injury.

Movement

Movements of the cervical spine include flexion, extension, lateral rotation, and lateral flexion. These movements are best seen from the side or front, and are expressed as a fraction of the usual range (Fig. 6.1). Restriction of movement occurs in arthritis and nerve compression.

Stressing

Stressing is not useful at the cervical spine.

Thoracic spine
Inspection

During inspection of the thoracic spine you should note any scoliosis (lateral fixed deviation) or kyphosis (anterior-facing concave curvature), which may be rounded or angular, due to collapsed vertebrae.

Palpation

During palpation, any tenderness of the thoracic spine can be due to collapse of T12 or L1 vertebrae, e.g. osteoporosis or trauma.

Movement

Movement of the thoracic spine is mainly rotational, but there is a small amount of flexion, extension, and lateral flexion (Fig. 6.2).

Stressing

Stressing is not useful at the thoracic spine.

Lumbosacral spine
Inspection

During inspection of the lumbosacral spine you should note any lordosis (posterior-facing concave curvature), scoliosis, vestigial ribs on the upper lumbar vertebrae, fusion of L5 with the sacrum (sacralization), and segmentation of S1 (lumbarization).

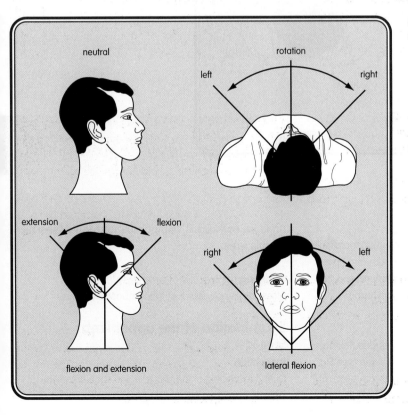

Fig. 6.1 Movements at the cervical spine.

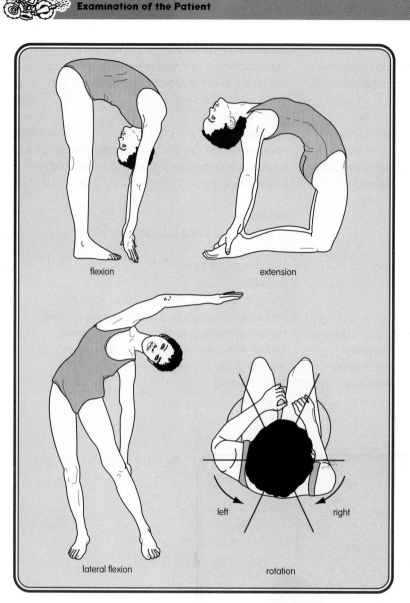

Fig. 6.2 Movements at the thoracic and lumbar spine.

flexion

extension

lateral flexion

left   right

rotation

Palpation

During palpation, any tenderness of the lumbosacral spine may be due to ligament strain, pain from disc prolapse with spinal canal narrowing and nerve compression, or perianal anaesthesia from a cauda equina lesion.

Movement

Movement of the lumbosacral spine includes flexion, extension, lateral rotation, and lateral flexion (see Fig. 6.2). Restriction follows different patterns, i.e. general restriction in osteoarthritis, asymmetrical flexion in disc

prolapse or scoliosis, and painful 'catch' on extension in muscle strain.

Stressing

Stressing is not useful at the lumbosacral spine.

Examination of the upper limb
Shoulder
Inspection

During inspection of the shoulder you should note its contour ('squaring off' in dislocation), swelling due to effusion (synovitis in subacromial bursa and glenohumeral joint), deltoid muscle wasting, winging of the scapulae (congenital or muscular dystrophies), alignment of the clavicle and acromion, and the way in which the arms are held (chronic conditions and pain may affect this).

Palpation

During palpation of the shoulder, tenderness and pain may be localized to different areas in the rotator cuff disorders. It may be due to glenohumeral or acromioclavicular arthritis, other arthropathies, or referred pain from other parts of the body.

Movement

Glenohumeral (abduction, adduction, flexion, extension, medial and lateral rotation) and scapular movements (elevation, retraction, and rotation) (Fig. 6.3) are possible at the shoulder. You should eliminate scapular

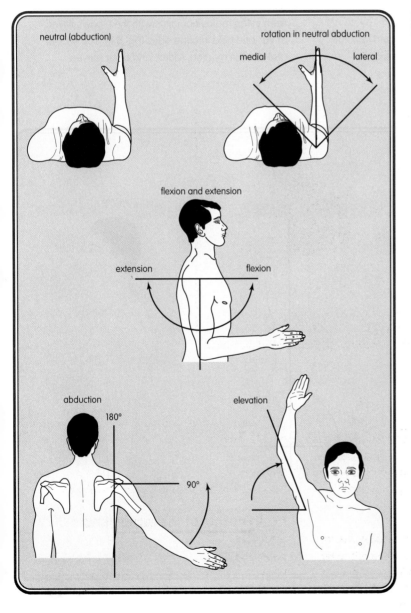

Fig. 6.3 Movements at the shoulder joint.

movement by pressing the scapula down at the top and asking the patient to move the shoulder. Check the power of deltoid (abduct the arm), serratus anterior (there is scapular 'winging' when both hands push firmly on a wall), and pectoralis major (push hands into waist). Check for abnormal movement between the acromion and the clavicle.

Stressing

Stressing is useful at the shoulder in checking for capsular lesions and osteoarthritis.

Elbow

Inspection

During inspection of the elbow you should look for 'gunstock' deformity (malunion of a previous supracondylar fracture), joint effusion swellings, soft lumps posteriorly (olecranon bursitis), and pebbly osteophytes (osteoarthritis).

Palpation

During palpation of the elbow you should note any tenderness of the lateral epicondyle ('tennis elbow'), medial epicondyle ('golfer's elbow'), and radial head (rheumatoid arthritis).

Movement

Flexion and extension movements are seen in the humero-ulnar joint; supination and pronation can be seen in the radioulnar joints with the elbows flexed at 90° and held into the sides (Fig. 6.4). You should also test the median, radial, and ulnar nerves.

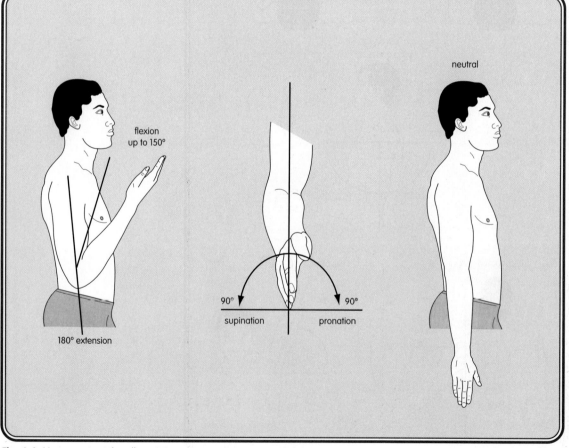

Fig. 6.4 Movements at the elbow joint.

Stressing
Stressing is not useful at the elbow.

Wrist
Inspection
During inspection of the wrist you should note any deformities or swellings of the tendon sheaths or joint capsule.

Palpation
During palpation of the wrist you should note any tenderness over the radial area (scaphoid fracture, de Quervain's tenosynovitis, osteoarthritis) or the ulnar area (tenosynovitis of extensors).

Movement
Flexion, extension, adduction, and abduction movements may be seen at the radiocarpal joint, and supination and pronation at the inferior radioulnar joints (Fig. 6.5).

Stressing
Stressing is not useful at the wrist.

Hands
Inspection
During inspection of the hands you should look for mallet finger, trigger finger, dropped finger, swan-neck or boutonnière deformities, a Z-deformity of the thumb,

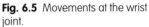

Fig. 6.5 Movements at the wrist joint.

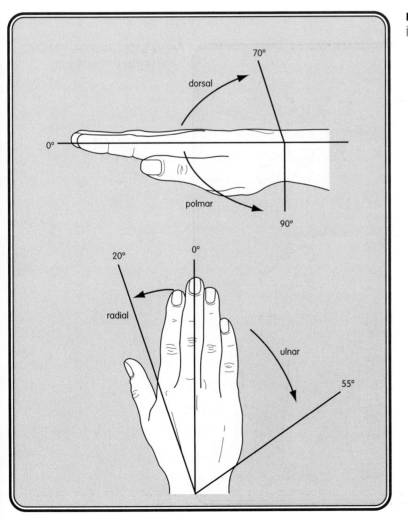

ulnar deviation of the fingers (rheumatoid arthritis), Heberden's nodes at the distal interphalangeal joint, Bouchard's nodes at the proximalinterphalangeal joints (osteoarthritis), ganglia, and thickening of the palmar aponeurosis (Dupuytren's contracture).

Palpation

During palpation of the hands you should note any tenderness over the anatomical snuffbox, indicating a fracture of the scaphoid; tender joints occur in rheumatoid arthritis.

Movement

Flexion, extension, adduction, and abduction movements can be seen at the metacarpophalangeal joints. There is also opposition of the thumb and little finger (Fig. 6.6). The interphalangeal joints only show flexion and extension.

Stressing

Stressing is useful at the hands—applying pressure on the fingers along their axis tests the mechanical stability of the metacarpals and phalanges.

Examination of the lower limb
Hip
Inspection

Inspection of the hip is not very useful, unless it involves watching the gait.

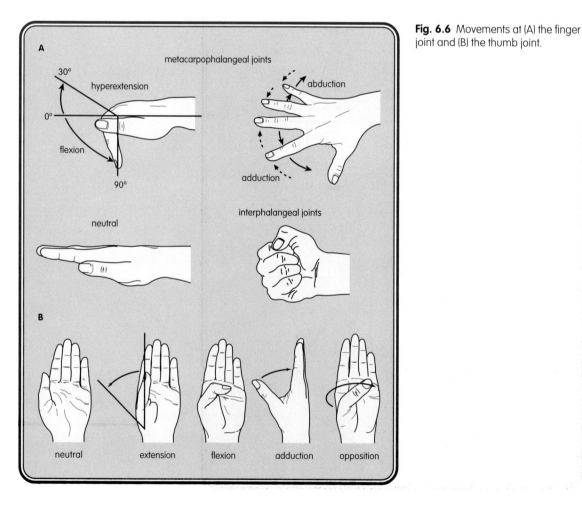

Fig. 6.6 Movements at (A) the finger joint and (B) the thumb joint.

Palpation

During palpation of the hip, you should note any pain at the front of the hip and the skin over the greater trochanter. You should measure the limbs to find their true length (from the anterior superior iliac spine to the medial malleolus, with the angle between the pelvis and limbs equal on both sides) or apparent length (from the xiphisternum to the medial malleolus, with the limbs lying parallel to the trunk).

Movement

Flexion, extension, abduction, adduction, medial rotation, and lateral rotation are possible at the hip (Fig. 6.7). You should note any fixed deformities which may be flexed, abducted, or adducted.

Stressing

Stressing is not very useful at the hip.

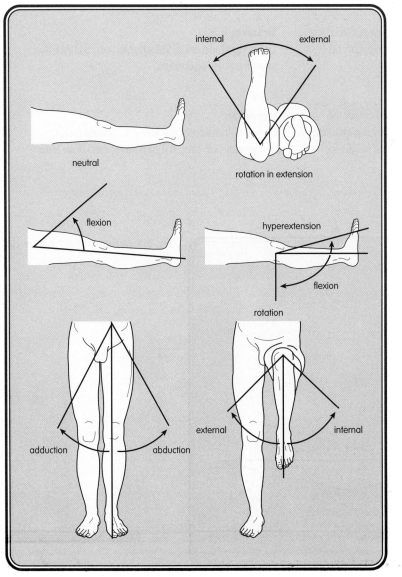

Fig. 6.7 Movements at the hip joint.

Knee

Inspection

During inspection of the knee you should look for genu valgum or genu varum, wasting of quadriceps femoris, and swelling around the knee (thickened bone or synovium, fluid within the joint, bursitis).

Palpation

During palpation of the knee you should note any tenderness over the joint due to torn menisci, synovitis, or osteoarthritis. Loose bodies may be felt in the suprapatellar region.

Movement

Flexion and extension movements are possible at the knee (Fig. 6.8). Many of these movements can be hyperextended.

Stressing

During stressing of the knee you should check the collateral ligaments in full extension and the cruciate ligaments with the knee flexed at a right angle.

Ankle

Inspection

During inspection of the ankle you should check the hypertrophic calf muscles to alert you to conditions such as Duchenne muscular dystrophy.

Palpation

During palpation of the ankle you should note any swelling near the joints that may indicate tenosynovitis.

Movement

Plantar flexion and dorsiflexion movements at the ankle are possible (Fig. 6.9). Inversion and eversion at the subtalar joint also occurs.

Stressing

Stressing of the ankle will enable you to check the integrity of the ligaments.

Feet

Inspection

During inspection of the feet you should look for congenital club foot, flat or hollow feet, claw toes,

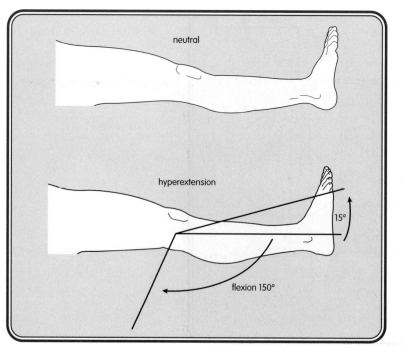

Fig. 6.8 Movements at the knee joint.

neutral

hyperextension

15°

flexion 150°

hammer toes, hallux valgus, hallux rigidus, bunions, calluses, and toenail lesions.

Palpation

During palpation of the feet you should check for a hot, swollen, first metatarsophalangeal joint. This is apparent in gout. You should also check the metatarsal heads for prominence and pain.

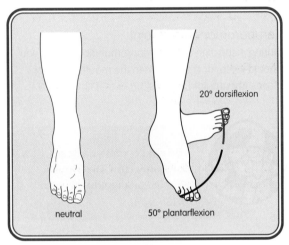

Fig. 6.9 Movements at the ankle joint.

Movement

Flexion and extension movements occur in the toes; inversion and eversion of the foot occurs at the midtarsal joint (Fig. 6.10).

Stressing

During stressing of the feet, longitudinal pressure will enable you to determine the integrity of the toes.

Examination of the thorax and abdomen

Thorax

Inspection

During inspection of the thorax you should look for deformities such as pectus carinatum (pigeon chest), pectus excavatum (funnel chest), scoliosis, and 'gibbus' (sharp angular deformity due to collapsed vertebrae from infection).

Palpation

During palpation of the thorax you should check for localized tenderness caused by broken ribs or metastasis.

Movement

Any restriction of expansion of the thorax to less than 5 cm is suggestive of ankylosing spondylitis.

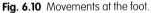

Fig. 6.10 Movements at the foot.

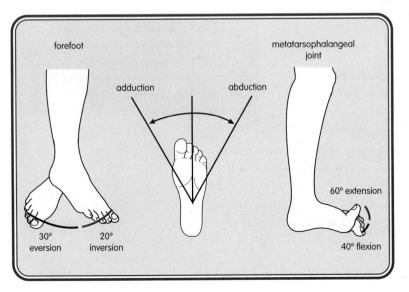

97

Stressing

During stressing of the thorax, lateral compression can cause pain if there is a broken rib.

Abdomen

Inspection

During inspection of the abdomen you should look for urethral discharge or balanitis (Reiter's syndrome).

Palpation

During palpation of the abdomen you should check for splenomegaly (Felty's syndrome), enlarged inguinal lymph nodes (rheumatoid arthritis), and renal enlargement (ankylosing spondylitis).

You should ask about bowel habit. A rectal and stool examination may be useful for the diagnosis of the enteropathic arthropathies, ulcerative colitis, and Crohn's disease.

Examination of the face

Eyes

During examination of the eyes you should check for any redness and dryness (Sjögren's syndrome), nodular scleritis and a thin blue sclera (rheumatoid arthritis), cataracts (steroid treatment for musculoskeletal disorders), iritis (ankylosing spondylitis), conjunctivitis (Reiter's syndrome), uveitis (Behçet's syndrome), and difficulty in closing the eyes (scleroderma).

Fundi

At the fundi, look for hyperviscosity (rheumatoid arthritis) or cytoid bodies composed of hard exudates [systemic lupus erythematosus (SLE)].

Mouth

At the mouth check for dryness and dental caries (Sjögren's syndrome), and ulcers (rheumatoid arthritis, SLE, Reiter's syndrome).

Facies

When examining the facies, check for parotid enlargement (Sjögren's syndrome), a cushingoid face (drugs used in rheumatoid arthritis and SLE), an expressionless, pinched 'bird-like' face (scleroderma), and alopecia (SLE and scleroderma).

Skin

You should check the skin for butterfly rash (SLE), urticaria and purpura (hypersensitive vasculitis in rheumatoid arthritis and SLE), malar telangiectasia, and skin tethering and pigmentation (scleroderma).

Temporomandibular joint

During inspection of the temporomandibular joint you should listen for crepitus when the mouth opens or closes (rheumatoid arthritis).

The chest, abdomen and face may also show signs of musculoskeletal disorders.

○ **Describe the normal appearance and range of movements possible at each specific joint.**
○ **Explain how to examine the back, shoulder, elbow, hand, hip, knee and feet for signs of musculoskeletal disorders.**

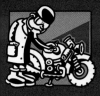

7. Further Investigations

Bone densitometry

Density of bone can be estimated by several techniques. These include:

- X-ray computerized tomography.
- Magnetic resonance imaging.
- Radioisotope scanning.

X-ray computerized tomography

X-ray computerized tomography (CT) involves X-ray scanning of part of the body from several angles and oscillators that detect the X-rays. Cross-sectional images are then compared and reconstructed by computer. These images can show variation in density between bone and surrounding tissue.

Magnetic resonance imaging (MRI).

In magnetic resonance imaging (MRI) scanning, the part of the body under investigation is placed in a magnetic field. Hydrogen nuclei (protons) are lined up in the direction of this magnetic field, assuming a new orientation when the electromagnetic radiation is altered. On stopping the radiation, the protons return to their original position and emit radiofrequency signals as they do so. It is these signals that can be analysed and converted into a two-dimensional image.

MRI scanning can detect variations in density of tissues. It provides a means of scanning without the use of X-rays.

Radioisotope scanning

During routine investigations using radioisotope scanning, an intravenous injection of radiolabelled technetium is administered. Rays emitted from the technetium can be measured with a gamma camera or rectilinear scanner.

As the isotope diffuses from bone matrix to blood, its increased uptake provides a measure of hyperaemia of bone and increased osteogenic activity.

Electromyography

Electromyography is a technique used to record the electrical activity in muscle both at rest and during contraction.

Method

During electromyography, a needle electrode is inserted into muscle. Electrical activity in the muscle is displayed on a cathode ray oscilloscope and heard on a speaker.

Electromyography is used:

- To determine whether a disorder is due to disease of the muscle or abnormalities of innervation.
- If there is an abnormality of innervation—this may be localized to the central nervous system, peripheral nerves, or neuromuscular junction.
- To aid in the diagnosis of myopathy, myotonia, and myasthenia.
- To obtain information about the distribution of a disorder so that a biopsy specimen can be taken from the appropriate site.
- To obtain information on the characteristics of motor units.

Assessment of muscle function

Normal muscle

Normal muscle at rest is electrically silent. The insertion of an electrode results in insertional activity because the muscle fibres are mechanically stimulated or damaged. If there is disease, the extent of this spontaneous activity may increase or decrease.

When insertional activity subsides, further activity may be seen only if the electrode is moved or the muscle contracts (Fig. 7.1).

Denervated muscle

Abnormal spontaneous activity of muscle at rest is termed fibrillation potentials. However, diseases of the neuromuscular junction and myopathies may also result in this pattern.

Myasthenia gravis

Single-fibre electromyography is used in the diagnosis of myasthenia gravis. This technique records the time

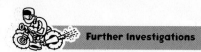

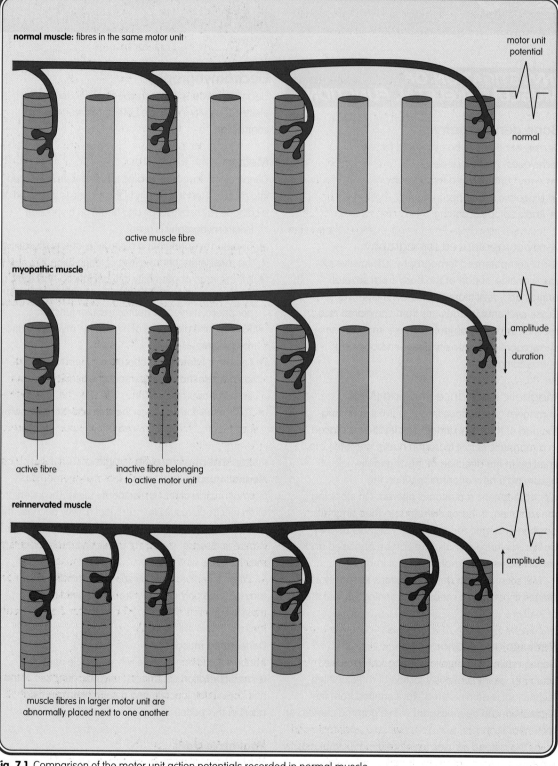

Fig. 7.1 Comparison of the motor unit action potentials recorded in normal muscle, myopathic muscle, and reinnervated muscle.

interval between the potentials of two fibres belonging to the same motor unit. In normal muscle this time interval is 10–50 µs but in myasthenia gravis it is increased.

Myopathic muscle
In myopathic muscle, the number of active muscle fibres in a motor unit is decreased (see Fig 7.1). This results in a reduced amplitude and action potential of shorter duration.

Reinnervated muscle
In reinnervated muscle, the muscle fibres are often reinnervated as a result of axonal sprouting of adjacent nerves (see Fig. 7.1). This results in a larger motor unit and therefore an increased amplitude of the recorded potential. In addition there is an unusual arrangement of fibres in the same unit, which may now lie next to each other.

Limitations
Electromyography does not provide a specific diagnosis, as certain types of recording may occur in more than one disorder. It is, therefore, always important to confirm a diagnosis with clinical findings and laboratory results.

Muscle biopsy
Method
Muscle samples are usually taken by needle biopsy. Local anaesthesia is required for this procedure.

An open biopsy may be needed in order to diagnose focal abnormalities such as myositis.

Evaluation
A muscle biopsy is usually evaluated in one or more ways, including:
- Histology.
- Histochemistry.
- Electron microscopy.
- Assays of enzyme activities.

With these techniques it is possible to assess muscle fibre types, the presence of inflammation or degeneration, the presence of abnormal mitochondria, and enzyme abnormalities.

Indications
Muscle biopsy differentiates between neuropathic and myopathic disorders. It is used to aid in the diagnosis of a range of inflammatory, dystrophic, and metabolic myopathies.

- List the techniques available to determine bone density.
- What are the uses and limitations of the EMG technique?
- Describe the technique of muscle biopsy.

ROUTINE INVESTIGATIONS IN MUSCULOSKELETAL DISORDERS

Haematology
Erythrocyte sedimentation rate
The erythrocyte sedimentation rate (ESR) is the rate at which red blood cells settle out of suspension in blood plasma in anticoagulated blood. A standard ESR tube is used and the length of clear plasma at the top of the settled blood cells is measured at one hour. The normal rate is <10 mm/h.

The ESR is raised in inflammatory conditions such as. rheumatoid arthritis, systemic lupus erythematosus (SLE), and inflammatory myopathy.

C-reactive protein
C-reactive protein is normally present in small amounts in serum, and is synthesized in greater amounts, by the liver, in response to a variety of insults, including infection.

C-reactive protein is raised in inflammatory conditions. It is a more sensitive indicator than ESR, but the results are not available as quickly.

Haemoglobin
Anaemia—usually normochromic, normocytic—occurs in inflammatory conditions such as rheumatoid arthritis and SLE.

White blood cell count
The numbers of white blood cells are raised in infections such as septic arthritis.

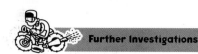

Thyroid function

The thyroid function test is able to exclude myopathy due to thyroid dysfunction; parathyroid hormone levels exclude myopathy associated with osteomalacia.

Blood biochemistry

Uric acid

Uric acid levels need be checked only if gout is suspected.

Muscle enzymes

Creatine kinase, a muscle enzyme, may be raised in inflammatory myopathy, muscular dystrophy, alcohol myopathy, and metabolic myopathy.

Bone enzymes

Alkaline phosphatase, a bone enzyme, is raised in Paget's disease, osteomalacia, and rickets, but not in osteoporosis.

Immunopathology

Autoantibodies

Autoantibodies that can be measured in musculoskeletal disorders include:

- Rheumatoid factor in rheumatoid arthritis, Sjögren's syndrome, SLE, polymyositis, dermatomyositis, and sarcoidosis.
- Antinuclear antibodies (ANA) in SLE (anti-Ro), Sjögren's syndrome, Still's disease, polymyositis (anti-Jo), and dermatomyositis.
- Anti-acetylcholine receptor in myasthenia gravis.

Synovial fluid analysis

Synovial fluid should be analysed for appearance, the presence of white blood cells and cultured for infections (Fig. 7.2).

- List the important blood tests in investigating the musculoskeletal system
- Describe the characteristics of synovial fluid found in osteoarthritis, rheumatoid arthritis and septic arthritis
- Be aware that crystals found in gout are negatively birefringent whereas in pseudogout they are positively birefringent

Synovial fluid changes in some rheumatic diseases				
Disease state	Appearance	White blood cells ($\times 10^6$/L)	Crystals	Culture
normal	clear viscous fluid	<200 mononuclear	none	sterile
osteoarthritis	increased volume; normal viscosity	3000 mononuclear	5% have pyrophosphate	sterile
rheumatoid arthritis	may be turbidly yellow or green; low viscosity	30 000 neutrophils	none	sterile
septic arthritis	turbid; low viscosity	50 000–100 000 neutrophils	none	positive
gout	clear; low viscosity	10 000 neutrophils	needle-shaped; negative birefringence	sterile
pyrophosphate arthropathy (pseudogout)	clear; low viscosity	10 000 neutrophils	brick-shaped; positive birefringence	sterile

Fig. 7.2 Synovial fluid changes in some rheumatic diseases. (Adapted with permission from *Clinical Medicine* 3rd edn, by P. Kumar and M. Clark, Baillière Tindall, 1994.).

IMAGING OF THE MUSCULOSKELETAL SYSTEM

The radiograph, or plain X-ray, is the imaging technique most commonly used to diagnose musculoskeletal disorders. It is simple, relatively cheap, and quick. However, in some instances, the radiograph may not yield sufficient information; then, other imaging techniques, such as MRI, CT, or radioisotope imaging, need to be employed.

Normal anatomy

The normal appearance of the musculoskeletal system during imaging is depicted in Figs 7.3 to 7.10. These include the:

- Skull (Fig. 7.3).
- Shoulder (Fig. 7.4).
- Elbow (Fig. 7.5).
- Hand (Fig. 7.6).
- Female pelvis (Fig. 7.7).
- Knee and leg (Fig. 7.8).
- Ankle (Fig. 7.9).
- Lumbar spine (Fig. 7.10).

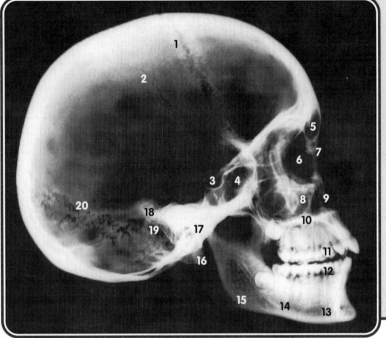

1	coronal suture
2	grooves for meningeal vessels
3	pituitary fossa
4	sphenoidal sinus
5	frontal sinus
6	orbit
7	nasal bones
8	maxillary sinus
9	anterior nasal spine
10	hard palate
11	maxilla and teeth
12	mandible and teeth
13	mental foramen
14	mandibular canal
15	angle of mandible
16	mastoid process
17	external acoustic meatus
18	petrous ridge
19	groove for sigmoid sinus
20	lamboid suture

Fig. 7.3 Lateral radiograph of skull. (Courtesy of Dr B. Berkovitz and Dr B. Moxham.)

1	Acromion process of scapula
2	Clavicle
3	Coracoid process of scapula
4	Head of humerus
5	Manubrium
6	Ribs
7	Spine of scapula

Fig. 7.4 Radiograph of the right shoulder. (Courtesy of Dr J. Calder and Dr G. Chessell.)

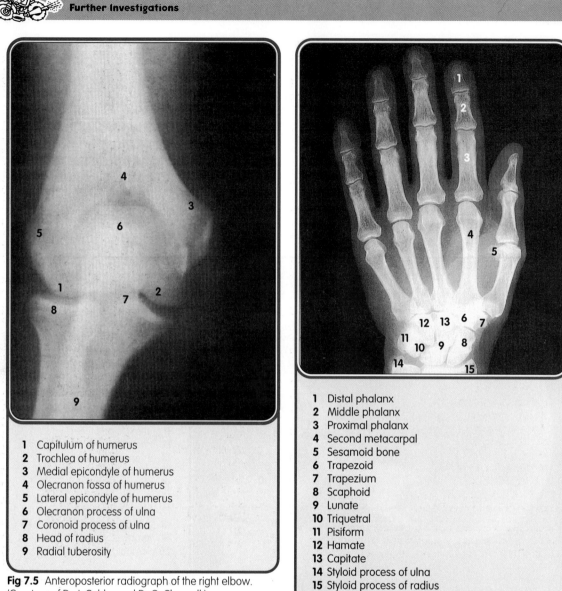

1   Capitulum of humerus
2   Trochlea of humerus
3   Medial epicondyle of humerus
4   Olecranon fossa of humerus
5   Lateral epicondyle of humerus
6   Olecranon process of ulna
7   Coronoid process of ulna
8   Head of radius
9   Radial tuberosity

Fig 7.5 Anteroposterior radiograph of the right elbow.
(Courtesy of Dr J. Calder and Dr G. Chessell.)

1   Distal phalanx
2   Middle phalanx
3   Proximal phalanx
4   Second metacarpal
5   Sesamoid bone
6   Trapezoid
7   Trapezium
8   Scaphoid
9   Lunate
10 Triquetral
11 Pisiform
12 Hamate
13 Capitate
14 Styloid process of ulna
15 Styloid process of radius

Fig 7.6 Radiograph of an adult hand. (Courtesy of Drs J.
Gosling, P. Harris, J. Humpherson, I. Whitmore, and P. Willan.)

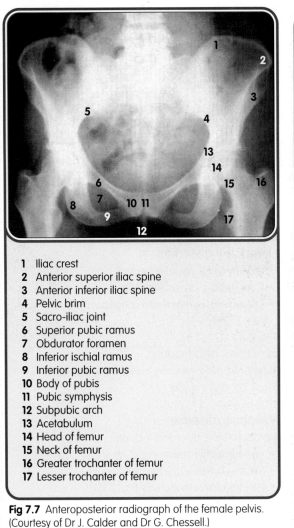

1 Iliac crest
2 Anterior superior iliac spine
3 Anterior inferior iliac spine
4 Pelvic brim
5 Sacro-iliac joint
6 Superior pubic ramus
7 Obdurator foramen
8 Inferior ischial ramus
9 Inferior pubic ramus
10 Body of pubis
11 Pubic symphysis
12 Subpubic arch
13 Acetabulum
14 Head of femur
15 Neck of femur
16 Greater trochanter of femur
17 Lesser trochanter of femur

Fig 7.7 Anteroposterior radiograph of the female pelvis.
(Courtesy of Dr J. Calder and Dr G. Chessell.)

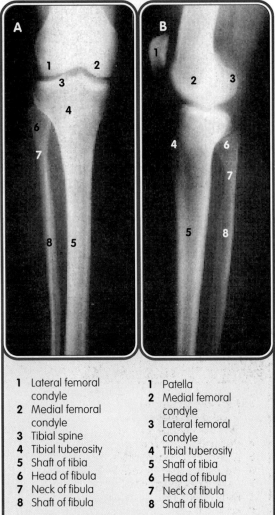

1 Lateral femoral condyle
2 Medial femoral condyle
3 Tibial spine
4 Tibial tuberosity
5 Shaft of tibia
6 Head of fibula
7 Neck of fibula
8 Shaft of fibula

1 Patella
2 Medial femoral condyle
3 Lateral femoral condyle
4 Tibial tuberosity
5 Shaft of tibia
6 Head of fibula
7 Neck of fibula
8 Shaft of fibula

Fig 7.8 Anteroposterior radiograph of (A) the right tibia and fibula. (B) Lateral radiograph of the right tibia and fibula.
(Courtesy of Dr J. Calder and Dr G. Chessell.)

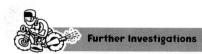
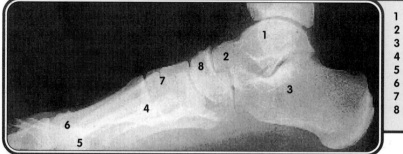

1	Medial malleolus
2	Head of talus
3	Calcaneus
4	Base of first metatarsal
5	Sesamoid bone
6	Head of first metatarsal
7	Cuneiforms
8	Navicular

Fig 7.9 Radiograph of the right foot and ankle showing longitudinal arches.
(Courtesy of Drs J. Gosling, P. Harris, J. Humpherson, I. Whitmore, and P. Willan.)

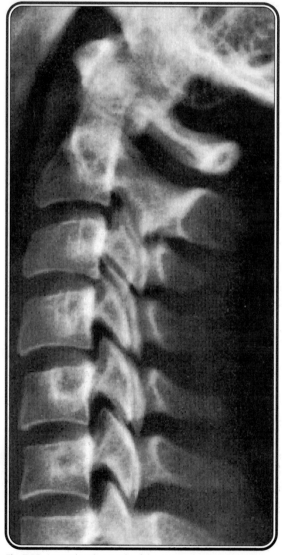

Fig 7.10 Lateral radiograph of the cervical spine. (Courtesy of Dr A. Greenspan and Dr P. Montesano.)

Bone disorders
Hereditary disorders
Hereditary bone disorders include:
- Congenital scoliosis (Fig. 7.11).
- Osteogenesis imperfecta congenita (Fig. 7.12).

Infections and trauma
Bone is prone to infection, called osteomyelitis (Fig. 7.13), and trauma.

Metabolic disease
Metabolic bone disorders include:
- Hyperparathyroidism (Fig. 7.14).
- Vitamin D deficiency (Fig. 7.15).
- Periarticular osteoporosis (Fig. 7.16).

Tumours
Hereditary bone tumours include:
- Osteosarcoma (Fig. 7.17).
- Giant-cell tumour (Fig. 7.18).

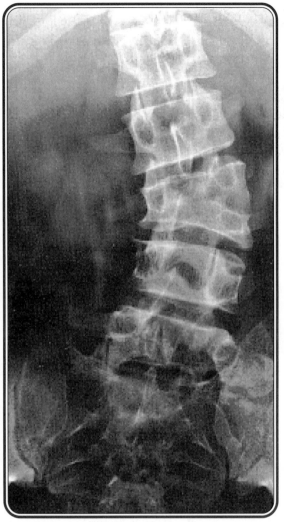

Fig. 7.11 Congenital scoliosis. This case of scoliosis in a 22-year-old man was due to hemivertebrae—a complete unilateral failure of formation. (Courtesy of Dr A. Greenspan.)

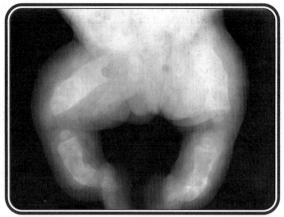

Fig. 7.12 Osteogenesis imperfecta congenita. This infant was born with type II osteogenesis imperfecta, where multiple fractures are present before birth. There is gross deformity of the lower limbs with multiple healing fractures. (Courtesy of Dr T. Lissauer.)

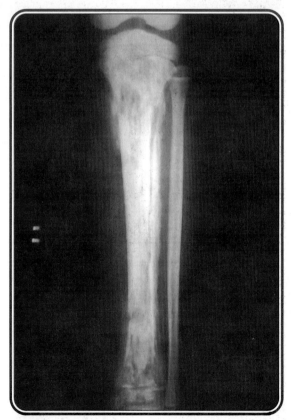

Fig. 7.13 Osteomyelitis. This chronic case shows a periosteal reaction along the lateral shaft of the tibia, and multiple hypodense areas within the metaphyseal region. (Courtesy of Dr T. Lissauer.)

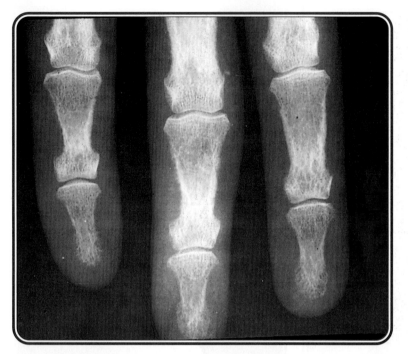

Fig. 7.14 Hyperparathyroidism. The terminal phalanxes show tufting and subperiosteal lesions, characteristic signs of primary hyperparathyroidism. (Courtesy of Dr P.M. Bouloux.)

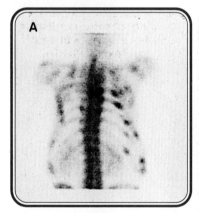

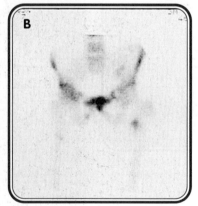

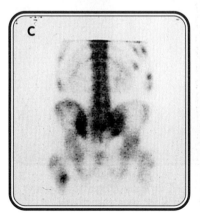

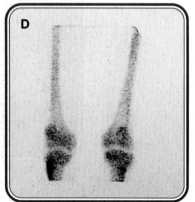

Fig. 7.15 Radioisotope bone scan showing a generalized increase in technetium uptake with multiple hot spots due to small fractures. The patient had metabolic bone disease due to vitamin D deficiency. The darker areas indicate increased uptake of technetium, representing altered cell growth. (A) thoracic spine, (B) pelvis, (C) lumbar spine, (D) Femur and knee joint. (Courtesy of Dr P.M. Bouloux.)

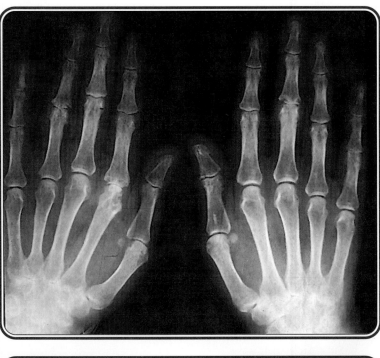

Fig. 7.16 Periarticular osteoporosis with mild ulnar changes in early rheumatoid arthritis. (Courtesy of Dr P.M. Bouloux.)

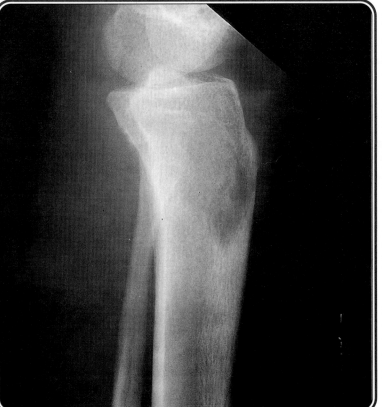

Fig. 7.17 Osteosarcoma in a child. The radiograph shows an infiltrative, poorly demarcated tumour in the metaphyseal region of the tibia. (Courtesy of Dr S. Taylor.)

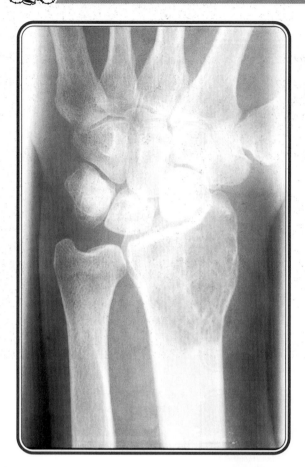

Fig. 7.18 Giant-cell tumour of the radius. Radiograph of the left wrist shows an expanding lytic lesion replacing the distal radius. The lesion is epiphyseal and abuts the adjacent articular surface. There is thinning of the radial cortex but no periosteal reaction and no reactive sclerosis at the proximal extent of the lesion. (Courtesy of Mr W.A. Jones.)

○ **Explain three ways of measuring bone density.**
○ **List some methods of assessing muscle function.**
○ **List routine laboratory investigations to assess musculoskeletal function.**
○ **Interpret normal radiographs of the skeleton.**
○ **Spot abnormalities in radiographs of diseased skeletons.**

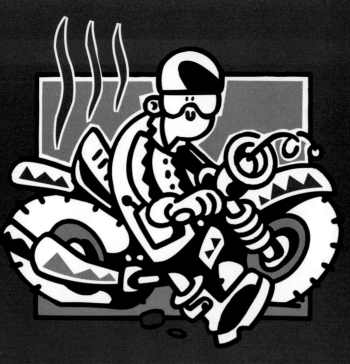

PATHOLOGY

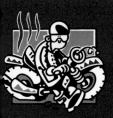

8. Pathology of Skeletal Muscle

Disorders of the neuromuscular junction (NMJ) can be classified into two types: presynaptic or postsynaptic. Both present with muscle weakness.

Presynaptic abnormalities
Botulism
Aetiology
Botulinum is an endotoxin produced by an organism called *Clostridium botulinum*.

Pathogenesis
Poisoning by botulinum is called botulism. Botulism is caused by the ingestion of canned meat contaminated with the endotoxin of *C. botulinum*.

The endotoxin acts by blocking the uptake of choline at the NMJ.

Clinical features
Botulism causes symmetrical descending paralysis, particularly of the face and respiratory muscles. Signs include diplopia, loss of pupillary reflex, and laryngeal palsy.

Diagnosis
The diagnosis of botulism is clinical and is confirmed by detection of the endotoxin in food or faeces.

Management
Management of botulism is by supportive care and antitoxin. Antibiotics may also be required.

Prognosis
There is an associated mortality of around 50% with botulism.

Lambert–Eaton myasthenic syndrome
The Lambert–Eaton myasthenic syndrome is a non-metastatic complication of malignancy that involves antibodies to voltage-gated Ca^{2+} channels in the presynaptic membrane.

Lambert–Eaton myasthenic syndrome is most often associated with small-cell lung carcinomas. The malignant cells express Ca^{2+} channels and may trigger the formation of the antibodies.

When nerves are stimulated at the NMJ, there is a decrease in Ca^{2+} influx. This leads to a decrease in the release of acetylcholine (ACh).

Patients with Lambert–Eaton myasthenic syndrome present with abnormal fatiguability.

Postsynaptic abnormalities
Myasthenia gravis
Epidemiology
Myasthenia gravis occurs most commonly in the third decade and has a male to female ratio of 1:2.

Aetiology
The cause of myasthenia gravis is unknown. It may be due to recurrent viral illness resulting in the formation of antibodies.

Pathology
Myasthenia gravis is an autoimmune disease (Fig. 8.1). In 90% of patients there are IgG antibodies to the ACh receptor in the postsynaptic membrane.

A decrease in functional ACh receptors results from:
- Stearic prevention of ACh binding to receptors due to the presence of antibody. The antibody does not itself bind to the ACh site, but prevents ACh from binding.
- Increased breakdown of receptors.

Clinical features
The main symptoms of myasthenia gravis are muscle weakness and fatiguability.

The ocular, bulbar, and cranial muscles are most commonly affected. Signs include ptosis and diplopia. There is generalized muscular weakness and the patient may be in respiratory distress. Muscle bulk is maintained until late in the disease.

Myasthenia gravis is remitting and relapsing, and is worse upon exercise.

Other autoimmune diseases, e.g. rheumatoid

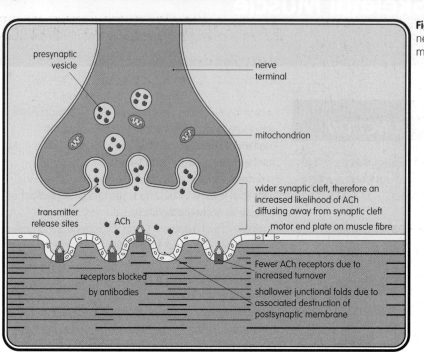

Fig. 8.1 Features of the neuromuscular junction in myasthenia gravis.

presynaptic vesicle

nerve terminal

mitochondrion

wider synaptic cleft, therefore an increased likelihood of ACh diffusing away from synaptic cleft

motor end plate on muscle fibre

transmitter release sites

ACh

receptors blocked by antibodies

Fewer ACh receptors due to increased turnover

shallower junctional folds due to associated destruction of postsynaptic membrane

arthritis and systemic lupus erythematosus (SLE), are often associated with myasthenia gravis. About 10% of patients have an associated thymoma and almost half of patients show thymic hyperplasia.

The heart is not affected.

Neonatal myasthenia may be seen in the newborn babies of mothers with the disease. The babies present with poor limb movements and poor feeding. These symptoms lasts a few weeks until the maternal antibodies decrease.

Diagnosis

About 90% of patients with myasthenia gravis have circulating anti-ACh receptor antibodies.

Diagnosis is based on the Tensilon test (Fig. 8.2). This test involves giving an injection of a short-acting anticholinesterase drug called edrophonium to the suspected myasthenic patient. As anticholinesterase drugs inhibit the enzyme acetylcholinesterase which hydrolyses ACh, thereby terminating the activation of ACh receptors on the muscle fibre, ACh is present in the synaptic cleft for longer and there is a greater probability that it will bind to the ACh receptor. In this way, muscle contraction can take place sufficiently for the patient to regain normal muscle strength temporarily.

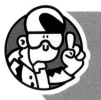

Understand myasthenia gravis because it is a common exam question.

An electromyogram (EMG) shows a decrease in response to stimulation.

Management

Management of myasthenia gravis is by the administration of long-lasting anticholinesterases, the dose varying according to the patient's response. Long-lasting anticholinesterases prolong the presence of ACh in the synaptic cleft, thereby increasing the likelihood of ACh binding to a receptor.

In those patients with an associated thymoma, thymectomy is needed.

Immunosupressives such as prednisolone or azathioprine are also useful.

Prognosis

The course of myasthenia gravis is variable. Death may result from aspiration pneumonia.

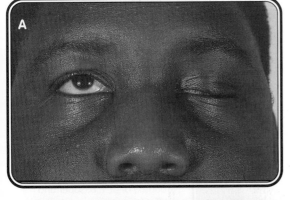

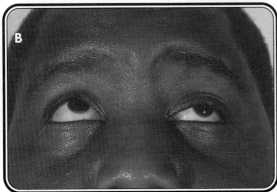

Fig. 8.2 The Tensilon test. (A) Muscle weakness caused by repeated facial movements. (B) There is rapid improvement after administration of edrophonium, a short-acting anticholinesterase. (Courtesy of Dr G.D. Perkin.)

> Disorders of the NMJ are not diseases of the muscle but rather disorders of function—hence atrophy tends to be a late feature.

> ○ Give examples of presynaptic and postsynaptic disorders of the NMJ.
> ○ What is myasthenia gravis?

INHERITED MYOPATHIES

Muscular dystrophies

The muscular dystrophies are a group of disorders involving a progressive degeneration of skeletal muscle.

X-linked dystrophies

Duchenne muscular dystrophy

Epidemiology

Duchenne muscular dystrophy occurs in 1 in 4000 live male births. One-third of the cases have no family history.

Spontaneous mutations are likely because the gene involved is large.

Aetiology

Duchenne muscular dystrophy is an X-linked recessive disorder.

Pathology

In Duchenne muscular dystrophy, a mutation occurs on the short arm of the X chromosome, the site (Xp21) coding for dystrophin protein. The lack of dystrophin protein results in impaired anchorage of muscle fibres to the extracellular matrix. This makes the muscle fibres more susceptible to tearing upon repeated contraction.

Damaged fibres allow an influx of calcium ions leading to irreversible cell death.

Clinical features

Children with Duchenne muscular dystrophy usually present at 2 years of age.

Symptoms include weakness of the pelvic and shoulder girdle muscles, and signs include selective atrophy, waddling gait, pseudohypertrophy of the calves, and Gower's sign (Fig. 8.3).

Diagnosis

The average age of diagnosis of Duchenne muscular dystrophy is 5 years.

Diagnosis is based on a raised serum creatinine phosphokinase concentration. Muscle biopsy also reveals necrosed muscle fibres surrounded by fibrous tissue and fat (Fig. 8.4). The muscle fibres are of variable diameters, owing to the body's attempt at regeneration.

115

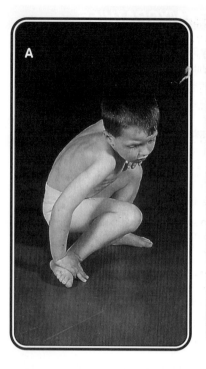
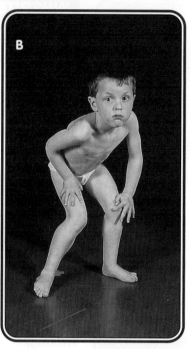

Fig. 8.3 Gower's sign showing the difficulty encountered in standing from the prone position in patients with Duchenne muscular dystrophy. (A) This child needs to turn prone to rise, then uses his hands to climb up on his knees. (B) Once at knee level the hands are released and the arms and trunk are swung sideways and upwards to reach an upright position. Note the hypertrophied calves (due to deposition of fat and fibrous tissue). (Courtesy of Dr T. Lissauer and Dr G. Clayden.)

muscle fbres
of varying size

connective
tissue

regenerating
fibres

Fig. 8.4 Histological changes in Duchenne muscular dystrophy showing variation in fibre diameter, increased fibrous and fatty connective tissue, and fibre generation.

Complications

Complications of Duchenne muscular dystrophy include marked scoliosis, impaired learning (30%), contractures, and cardiomyopathy.

Management

There is no treatment that will halt Duchenne muscular dystrophy; management is supportive and is aimed at maintaining the use of the muscles and decreasing respiratory symptoms.

Identification of female carriers is possible and genetic counselling may be offered.

Prognosis

Most people with Duchenne muscular dystrophy are wheelchair bound by their teens. Death occurs in the late teens or the early twenties, due to cardiac failure or failure of the respiratory muscles.

Becker muscular dystrophy

Becker muscular dystrophy is a less common X-linked variant of Duchenne muscular dystrophy. It shows similar clinical features to Duchenne muscular dystrophy, although the progression of the disease is slower. The average age of onset is 11 years with death occurring in the 40s.

Autosomal dystrophies

Limb girdle dystrophy

Limb girdle dystrophy, one of the autosomal recessive dystrophies, presents in childhood or adult life with pelvic and shoulder girdle weakness (Fig. 8.5).

Pseudohypertrophy of the calves is less common than that in Duchenne muscular dystrophy.

Muscle biopsy shows findings similar to those of Duchenne muscular dystrophy.

Prognosis involves a variable degree of disability.

Facioscapulohumeral dystrophy

Facioscapulohumeral dystrophy is an autosomal dominant disorder. The condition presents in childhood or adult life with face and shoulder girdle weakness. Winging of the scapulae is characteristic.

Pseudohypertrophy is rare.

Muscle biopsy shows findings similar to those of Duchenne muscular dystrophy.

Individuals show a mild degree of disability.

Myotonic disorders

Myotonic disorders are a group of conditions in which there is a delay in muscle relaxation after voluntary contraction. Administration of general anaesthetics is more likely to cause complications in patients with muscle disorders of this sort.

Myotonic dystrophy

Epidemiology

Myotonic dystrophy occurs in 1 in 8000 people.

Aetiology

Myotonic dystrophy is an autosomal dominant disorder.

Pathology

Myotonic dystrophy is caused by a mutation on chromosome 19, the site coding for a cAMP-dependent kinase.

In affected families the disease is more severe in later generations. This is known as anticipation.

Clinical features

Myotonic dystrophy may occur in the newborn period with hypotonia. More commonly, it presents in the early

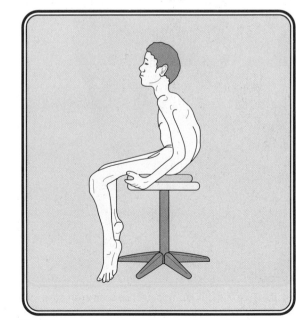

Fig. 8.5 Severe limb girdle dystrophy demonstrating proximal muscle wasting and kyphosis.

20s, with limb weakness, distal wasting, characteristic facies, and cranial muscle involvement (Fig. 8.6). Learning difficulties may also be present.

Other associated findings include cataracts, baldness, gonadal atrophy, and glucose intolerance.

Diagnosis
Diagnosis of myotonic dystrophy is mainly clinical, although an EMG is characteristic.

A muscle biopsy shows dystrophic changes.

Management
The management of myotonic dystrophy involves treating the myotonia, although this does not influence the course of the disease.

Prognosis
Death from myotonic dystrophy is usually due to cardiomyopathy or involvement of the respiratory muscles.

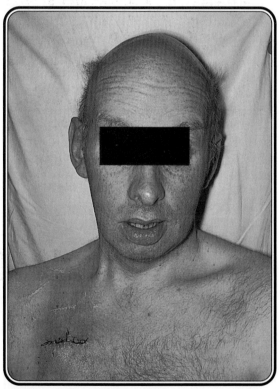

Fig. 8.6 Typical 'monk like' appearance seen in an adult with myotonic dystrophy. Note the facial weakness, atrophy of temporal and sternocleidomastoid muscles, and frontal baldness. (Courtesy of Dr G.D. Perkin.)

Congenital myotonia
Congenital myotonia, or Thomsen's disease, is a rare disorder that may be dominant or recessive. Symptoms include myotonia—this is worse in cold temperatures and with rest.

Generalized muscle hypertrophy is prominent.

Paramyotonia congenita
Paramyotonia congenita is an autosomal dominant condition. The mutation occurs on chromosome 17, the site coding for the sodium channel.

Paramyotonia congenita is a non-progressive muscle weakness that is worse in cold temperatures.

Metabolic myopathies
The metabolic myopathies are a heterogenous group of conditions in which there are abnormalities in muscle energy metabolism.

Primary metabolic myopathies
Glycogen storage disorders
Glycogen storage disorders are caused by enzyme anomalies inherited in a recessive manner.

The degree of muscle involvement is variable between the major types of primary metabolic myopathies.

Symptoms arise as a result of the decreased availability of energy from glycolysis. This is due to an impaired ability to mobilize glucose from glycogen.

Glycogen storage disorder type V (McArdle's syndrome) is an autosomal recessive disorder in which there is a deficiency of skeletal muscle myophosphorylase. Symptoms include temporary weakness and muscle cramps on exercise. There is an associated myoglobinuria. There is no rise in venous lactate during exercise, which aids diagnosis by enzyme analysis of muscle tissue. Life expectancy is not affected. Patients are advised to avoid exercise.

Lipid disorders
In the lipid disorders, there is a decreased availability of energy to muscle due to abnormalities in fatty acid metabolism.

Patients usually present with hypotonia in infancy or muscle weakness and cramps later.

Symptoms are worse with prolonged exercise or fasting.

Mitochondrial disorders

The mitochondrial disorders are inherited. These are abnormalities of either the mitochondrial genome (more commonly) or the nuclear genome.

The age of onset is variable. The muscle weakness (particularly of the extraocular muscles) may be isolated or associated with neurological and metabolic disturbances.

Muscle biopsy shows abnormal mitochondria with crystalline inclusions.

Mitochondrial myopathy may develop in patients on long-term zidovudine therapy, i.e. patients infected with HIV.

Secondary metabolic myopathies

Myopathic symptoms can occur as a result of a whole range of electrolyte disturbances, e.g. Ca^{2+}, Mg^{2+}, K^+ etc.

Endocrine disorders are examples of secondary metabolic myopathies which are acquired (p. 135).

Periodic paralyses

The periodic paralyses are a rare group of disorders characterized by repeated attacks of muscle weakness.

There are three types—hypokalaemic, hyperkalaemic, and normokalaemic.

Hypokalaemic periodic paralysis

Hypokalaemic periodic paralysis is an autosomal dominant condition. It presents in adolescence and is remitting in the late 30s.

Attacks often occur after strenuous exercise or a heavy carbohydrate meal. During an attack, the serum potassium concentration is low (2.5–3.5 mmol/L)—attacks are terminated by the administration of intravenous potassium chloride.

Diuretic therapy and thyrotoxicosis must be excluded as possible causes of the myopathy.

Hyperkalaemic periodic paralysis

Hyperkalaemic periodic paralysis is an autosomal dominant condition. It presents in childhood and is remitting in the 20s.

Attacks may occur after strenuous exercise and are terminated by intravenous calcium gluconate. During an attack the serum potassium concentration is high (6–7 mmol/L).

Attacks last for a shorter period than those associated with hypokalaemia.

Normokalaemic periodic paralysis

Normokalaemic periodic paralysis is a very rare condition. The attacks respond to sodium.

Of the inherited myopathies, Duchenne muscular dystrophy is a common topic in exams.

- Describe a simple classification of the inherited myopathies.
- Describe Duchenne muscular dystrophy and give a differential diagnosis.
- Describe the clinical features of myotonic dystrophy.
- Give examples of metabolic myopathies.
- List the three types of periodic paralyses.

ACQUIRED MYOPATHIES

Idiopathic inflammatory myopathies

The idiopathic inflammatory myopathies are uncommon disorders and have a male:female ratio of 1:2.

Most people with idiopathic inflammatory myopathy present in middle age.

Polymyositis

Polymyositis is the most common inflammatory myopathy.

Aetiology

The cause of polymyositis is not known, although it may be autoimmune in origin. A viral cause (coxsackie virus) has been suggested.

Polymyositis is a non-metastatic complication of malignancy, as more than 10% of patients have an underlying malignancy that presents later, e.g. carcinoma of the breast, bronchus, or gastrointestinal tract. In this instance the male to female ratio is reversed.

Pathology

In polymyositis there is inflammation and destruction of both type I and type II muscle fibres due to the action of cytotoxic T lymphocytes. Histologically there is fibre necrosis, muscle atrophy, and evidence of fibre regeneration.

Clinical features

There is progressive, symmetrical, proximal muscle weakness in polymyositis. The respiratory and heart muscles may also be affected. Dysphagia and dysarthria are other features.

Polymyositis is associated with other connective tissue diseases such as SLE and rheumatoid disease. Features typical of connective tissue diseases may be present, e.g. Raynaud's phenomenon, in which there is intermittent vasospasm of arterioles in the hands and feet in response to cold and emotional stimuli. It is usually painful and the affected part of the body goes through the following colour change: pale–blue–red.

Diagnosis

The diagnosis of polymyositis involves two of three findings:
- Raised serum creatine phosphokinase concentrations.
- A characteristic EMG.
- A muscle biopsy.

Antinuclear antibodies (Jo-1) and rheumatoid factor may also be present.

Management

The management of polymyositis includes immunosupressive drugs (causing remission), and physiotherapy to prevent disuse atrophy of muscles.

Underlying malignancy must be excluded.

Prognosis

The course of polymyositis is variable.

Death results from aspiration pneumonia and respiratory or heart failure.

Dermatomyositis

Dermatomyositis is closely related to polymyositis, sharing features previously described.

In addition to muscular symptoms there are associated skin changes:
- A characteristic purple heliotrope rash, usually on the eyelids, although it may spread to other sites.
- An erythematous rash on the face, scalp, shoulders, and hands.

Inclusion body myositis

Inclusion body myositis affects mainly the elderly and is clinically similar to polymyositis.

Electron microscopy demonstrates the presence of filamentous inclusions in the muscle fibres.

It is a progressive disorder and immunosuppressive therapy is not as effective.

Endocrine myopathies (or secondary metabolic myopathies)

Corticosteroid-induced myopathy

Corticosteroid-induced myopathy is caused by an excess of corticosteroid, e.g. Cushing's syndrome or people on steroid therapy.

The myopathy is proximal, i.e. it affects the upper parts of the arms and legs.

There is a raised creatine kinase concentration, and muscle biopsy reveals selective atrophy of type II muscle fibres.

Myopathy of thyroid dysfunction

Thyrotoxicosis may be associated with a proximal myopathy.

Hypothyroidism may result in symptoms of muscle stiffness and a proximal myopathy.

Myopathy of osteomalacia

All causes of osteomalacia (e.g. vitamin D deficiency, liver failure, liver enzyme-inducing drugs) may result in a proximal myopathy.

Toxic myopathies

Toxic myopathies are caused by excess alcohol or drugs.

Excess alcohol

In toxic myopathy, caused by excess alcohol, two patterns of myopathy are seen:

- Subacute proximal myopathy (which may be reversed in the early stages); this is seen in chronic alcoholics. Selective atrophy of type II muscle fibres occurs.
- Acute myopathy associated with severe muscle pain due to acute alcohol excess—myoglobinuria may also occur.

Drug-induced myopathies

Agents that may cause a subacute proximal myopathy include cholesterol-lowering agents, (e.g. benzofibrate), as well as chloroquine, penicillamine, and lithium. Patients respond to removal of the drug.

Viral myalgias

The viral myalgias are muscle weakness associated with a viral illness, usually respiratory.

Myalgic encephalomyelitis (ME; also known as postviral/chronic fatigue syndrome or 'yuppie flu') is a disorder in which the patient presents with muscular fatigue and pain on movement. The cause is unknown and other associated symptoms include poor concentration and depression. The disorder tends to affect women and opinions differ as to whether this is a psychological or a skeletal muscle disorder.

Endocrine and toxic causes of myopathy are useful to remember as they can be easily included on a list of differential diagnosis for myopathy

○ **Give a simple classification of the main acquired myopathies.**

9. Pathology of Bone

HEREDITARY ABNORMALITIES OF BONE

Osteogenesis imperfecta

Osteogenesis imperfecta, or brittle bone disease, is a group of disorders that are inherited in several ways and have varying degrees of severity (Fig. 9.1). The genes responsible for osteogenesis imperfecta are found on chromosomes 7 and 17. The incidence of osteogenesis imperfecta is 1 in 20 000.

Pathology

In osteogenesis imperfecta, there is an abnormal synthesis of type I collagen that makes up 90% of bone matrix. Some forms of the disorder are fatal in the perinatal period; others predispose to fractures but there is overall survival.

Morphology

Osteopenia (decreased bone) occurs in osteogenesis imperfecta. This involves thinning of the cortex and trabeculae.

Other features

Other features of osteogenesis imperfecta include uveal pigment (blue) that can be seen through thin sclerae, deafness, and dental abnormalities.

Osteopetrosis

Osteopetrosis, also known as Albers–Schöenberg or marble bone disease, is a group of rare inherited disorders of different severities (Fig. 9.2). If the condition is autosomal recessive it presents from birth as anaemia, leucocytopenia, and sometimes death. Adult types predispose to fractures.

Pathology

Osteopetrosis is a defect in osteoclast function leading to decreased bone resorption and net bone overgrowth.

Morphology

In osteopetrosis there is overgrowth and sclerosis of bone, marked thickening of cortex, and narrowing and filling of medullary cavity (inhibits haemopoiesis). Treatment is with marrow transplant.

Achondroplasia

Achondroplasia is also known as dwarfism. It is a disorder caused by a single gene inherited in an autosomal dominant manner with complete penetrance. The incidence of achondroplasia is 1 in 25 000.

Homozygotes die soon after birth, whereas heterozygotes have a normal lifespan and normal mental, sexual, and reproductive development.

Pathology

In achondroplasia there is derangement of endochondral ossification.

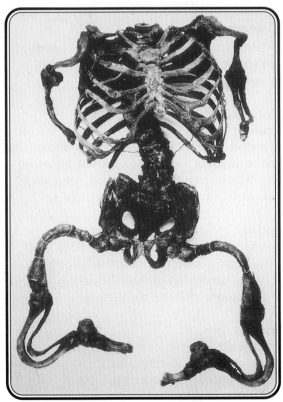

Fig. 9.1 Skeleton of a child with osteogenesis imperfecta congenita. Note the deformed limbs, scoliosis, and chest and pelvic deformities. (Courtesy of Dr P.G. Bullough and Dr V.J. Vigorita.)

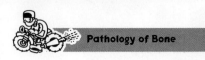

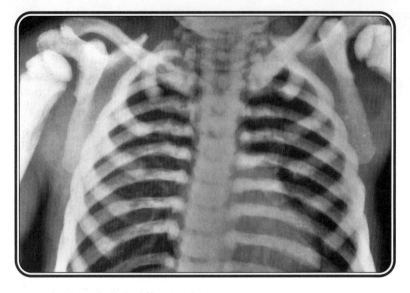

Fig. 9.2 Radiograph of the upper body of a child with osteopetrosis, showing a marked increase in density of all the bones. (Courtesy of Dr P.G. Bullough and Dr V.J. Vigorita.)

Morphology

Achondroplastic heterozygotes have short limbs and a normal-sized trunk. The skull is enlarged and there is a big forehead and depression of the nasal bridge. The epiphyses are abnormally wide (appositional growth is unaffected).

Malformations

Occasionally, malformations of the bones in the skeleton occur in achondroplasia. These result from either:

- Failure of formation.
- Extra bones (in fingers and toes).
- Fusion of bones (skull sutures).

Generally, these malformations are of no consequence. However, correction is possible for cosmetic reasons.

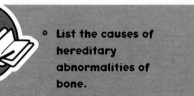

○ List the causes of hereditary abnormalities of bone.

INFECTIONS AND TRAUMA

Osteomyelitis

Osteomyelitis, or infection of bone, can be caused by any bacterial agent, especially in people who are immunosuppressed (Fig. 9.3).

Pyogenic osteomyelitis

Causes

In immunocompromised people, pyogenic osteomyelitis can be caused by *Staphylococcus aureus, Escherichia coli, Klebsiella* spp., *Pseudomonas* spp., salmonellae, *Haemophilus influenzae*, and *Streptococcus* spp.

Spread

Spread of infection into bone can be by blood, local tissues, open fracture, or surgery. In developing countries, spread is usually haematogeneous, whereas in developed countries it is due to trauma.

Histology

Infection of bone leads to ischaemic necrosis, fibrosis, and bony repair. Necrosis of a bone segment is known as a sequestrum. This is surrounded by a sheath of subperiosteal new bone called the involucrum. Very sclerotic new bone forms a pattern called Garré's sclerosing osteomyelitis. There may be formation of sinus

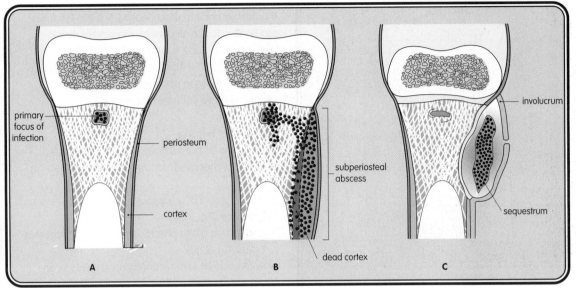

Fig. 9.3 Sequence of osteomyelitis. The primary focus of infection (A) has spread through bone, causing the death of cortical bone, and formation of a subperiosteal abcess (B). Death of a segment of bone (sequestrium) occurs (C), and the area is surrounded by new subperiosteal bone (involucrum)

tracts or abscesses called Brodie's abscesses (these are sometimes sterile).

Clinical features
Infection of bone causes acute bone pain and fever. The infection usually starts in the metaphysis, where the good blood supply encourages bacterial growth and enables spread to other areas. A lytic area surrounded by a zone of reactive new bone can be seen on radiographs.

Complications
Complications of bone infection include sinus tracts to the skin surface (called cloacae), fracture, septicaemia, endocarditis, pyogenic arthritis, and an alteration in growth rate.

Tuberculous osteomyelitis
Tuberculous osteomyelitis is relatively uncommon in people who are immunocompetent. About 2% of all cases of tuberculosis have bone involvement.

Spread
Tuberculous osteomyelitis is spread haematogenously. It is more destructive and resistant to control than the pyogenic form.

Clinical features
Tuberculous osteomyelitis is usually a chronic condition with involvement of a single bone (except in AIDS). It occurs in long bones, and in the thoracic and lumbar vertebrae, where it is called Pott's disease.

Complications
Tuberculous osteomyelitis causes fractures, nerve compression, and tuberculous arthritis.

Syphilis
Syphilis in the skeleton
Syphilis of bone can be either congenital or acquired (Fig. 9.4). The condition is rare because of its early treatment with penicillin.

Histology
In syphilis of bone, local periostitis leads to new bone formation on the outer cortex. Gummata are the characteristic lesions of syphilis. They have a centre of rubbery, grey–white coagulation necrosis surrounded by epitheloid or fibroblastic cells.

Clinical features
On radiographs of affected skulls, the effects of syphilis are seen as a 'crew-cut' outline. When the tibia is

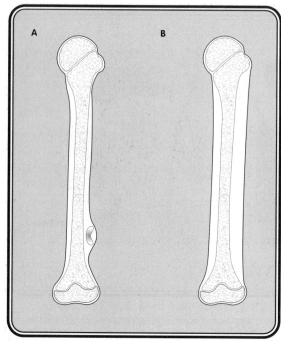

Fig. 9.4 Syphilis in bone showing (A) localized and (B) diffuse bone thickening.

involved there is a 'sabre shin' appearance. The destruction and collapse of nasal and parietal bones can create a 'saddle nose'.

Fractures
Types
There are several types of bone fractures. These are:
- Simple (clean break).
- Comminuted (multiple bone fragments).
- Compound (break through overlying skin).
- Stress (small linear fragments).
- Pathological (bones weakened by disease).

Causes
Fractures are usually caused by trauma, which is either substantial or minor and repeated. Pathological fractures arise from diseases, e.g. tumours, osteoporosis, Paget's disease, osteomalacia.

Healing
Healing of fractures requires immobilization of approximated bone ends and good alignment.

Delayed or imperfect healing
The delayed or imperfect healing of bone fractures can be due to malalignment, movement during healing, poor blood supply, and soft tissue interposition in the fracture gap. Either can occur in the elderly, those in poor general health, and in people who are immunosuppressed.

Histology of healing
Healing of a fracture follows a sequence (Fig. 9.5). The histological changes that take place during healing include:
- Development of a haematoma, which forms a soft procallus (Fig. 9.5A).
- Conversion of the procallus to a fibrocartilaginous callus (Fig. 9.5B).
- Replacement of fibrocartilaginous callus to an osseous callus—trabecular lamellar bone (Fig. 9.5C,D).
- Remodelling along weightbearing lines by osteoclasts (Fig. 9.5E).

Complications
Complications of fractures can include malunion of bones, avascular necrosis, shock, osteoarthritis, infection, and deep vein thrombosis.

Avascular necrosis
Pathology
Avascular necrosis involves the death of bone and marrow without infection, and is due to a poor blood supply. It is mostly seen in the head of femur and scaphoid, occurring when fractures deprive adjacent areas of their blood supply (Fig. 9.6). Medullary infarctions affect cancellous bone and bone marrow, with cortical sparing. Subchondral infarctions lead to wedge-shaped areas of damage.

Causes
Avascular necrosis can be idiopathic or caused by trauma, thrombo-embolism, sickle-cell disease, polycythaemia, immunosuppression, or decompression sickness (divers).

Histology
Dead bone is identified by empty lacunae surrounded by necrotic adipocytes. The adipocytes may rupture to

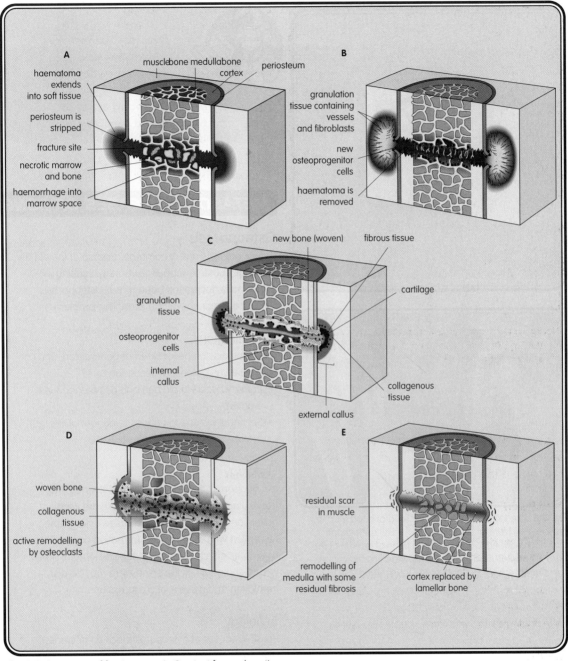

Fig. 9.5 Sequence of fracture repair. See text for explanation.

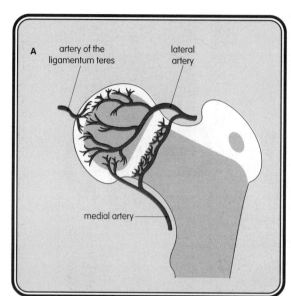

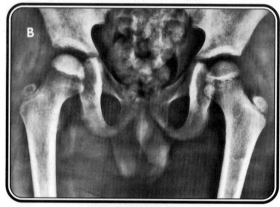

Fig. 9.6 Avascular necrosis of the femoral head (Perthe's disease). (A) Normal blood supply, and (B) radiograph showing widened joint space, cessation of growth of the bony epiphyses, and increased growth of cartilage. (Courtesy of Dr P.G. Bullough and Dr V.J. Vigorita.)

release fatty acids, which bind calcium and form deposits. There is osteoclastic resorption of trabeculae and the articular cartilage is distorted.

Clinical features

There is pain and immobility in avascular necrosis—the patient cannot walk, especially if the condition is a complication of fracture (elderly).

○ **Describe the features of osteomyelitis, particularly the pyogenic type.**
○ **List the different types of fracture and how they heal.**

METABOLIC DISEASES OF BONE

Osteoporosis

Osteoporosis is a very common disease of the elderly, especially postmenopausal women, resulting in abnormally decreased bone mass. Osteoporosis causes a major social and economic problem.

Classification

Osteoporosis can be localized or generalized, and can be classed as primary or secondary:

- Primary occurs in old age and postmenopausal women.
- Secondary is due to endocrine abnormalities, gut malabsorption, and neoplasia.

Histology

In osteoporosis the bone cortex has thinned, the trabeculae are attenuated, and there are wide haversian canals (Fig. 9.7). Increased osteoclastic resorption with slowed bone formation occurs. The main sites affected are the vertebrae, femoral necks, wrists, and pelvis. In the spine there may be disc herniation and nerve root compression.

Aetiology

Possible causes of osteoporosis include decreased exercise; oestrogen deficiency; lack of calcium, vitamin D or fluoride; hyperadrenocorticism; hypogonadism;, thyrotoxicosis; hypopituitarism; pregnancy; immobilization; diabetes; and long-term heparin administration.

Clinical features

Osteoporosis causes bone pain, loss of height, fractures, and deformities such as lumbar lordosis and

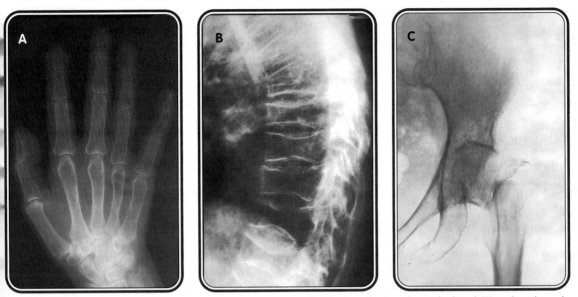

Fig. 9.7 Features of osteoporosis. (A) Loss of cortical thickening and reduction of trabeculae in the hand, (B) wedge-shaped flattening of vertebral bodies leading to loss of height, and (C) fracture of the neck of the femur in an elderly person. (Courtesy of Dr P.G. Bullough and Dr V.J. Vigorita.)

kyphoscoliosis. Diagnosis is by bone density scans or biopsy. A 30% loss of bone mass is required before radiographs show translucency.

Treatment for osteoporosis includes hormone replacement to increase oestrogen levels, and exercise to strengthen weightbearing joints.

Rickets and osteomalacia

Rickets occurs in growing children and osteomalacia in adults. These are caused by either vitamin D deficiency or phosphate depletion—the latter is less common.

Aetiology

Vitamin D deficiency can be caused by low quantities in the diet, insufficient exposure to sunlight, malabsorption, or deranged liver or kidney metabolism. Phosphate depletion can be caused by X-linked phosphataemia, neoplasia, or poisoning from heavy metals.

Pathology

Rickets and osteomalacia arise from a failure of bone mineralization, which leads to softer and wider channels of matrix. Excess unmineralized matrix and underdeveloped epiphyseal cartilage calcification leads to endochondral bone that is deranged and overgrown.

Clinical features

Rickets presents with bowing of the legs, overgrowth of costochondral junctions (forming a 'rachitic rosary'), widened epiphyses, and either a flattened ('bossed') square skull or craniotabes (the skull snaps back into shape after being pressed in) (Fig. 9.8).

Osteomalacia presents with spontaneous incomplete fractures ('Looser's zones') in long bones and the pelvis, bone pain, weakened proximal limb muscles, and a decreased serum calcium.

Bone biopsy is needed to confirm the diagnosis of rickets or osteomalacia. Treatment involves vitamin D administered orally or intravenously, and an improved diet.

Hyperparathyroidism

Classification

Hyperparathyroidism can be either:

- Primary—due to a lesion of the parathyroid gland which increases parathyroid hormone (PTH) (raised serum calcium) levels.

129

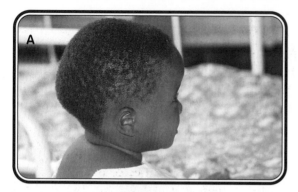

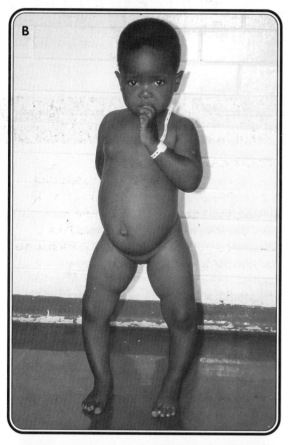

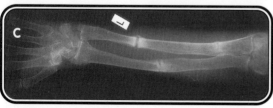

Fig. 9.8 Rickets and osteomalacia. (A) Skull 'bossing' in rickets, (B) lateral and forward bowing of legs in rickets, and (C) radiograph showing pseudofractures (Looser's zones) in the forearm in osteomalacia. (A and B courtesy of Dr S. Taylor and Dr A. Raffles; C courtesy of Dr P.G. Bullough and Dr V.J. Vigorita.)

- Secondary—due to bone metastases, inappropriate PTH secretion by tumours, or renal failure (normal or lowered serum calcium).

Pathology

In hyperparathyroidism, increased PTH levels cause an increase in osteoclast activity that leads to increased bone resorption.

Histology

In hyperparathyroidism, demineralization leads to increased osteoclast activity and resorption. There is characteristic peritrabecular fibrosis, called osteitis fibrosa, and more marked fibrosis and cyst formation within the marrow (osteitis fibrosa cystica or von Recklinghausen's disease of the bone). 'Brown tumours' of osteoclasts, fibrosis, and haemorrhage are also seen (Fig. 9.9). These resemble giant-cell granulomas.

Clinical features

In hyperparathyroidism, radiographs of the phalanges and clavicles show 'moth-eaten' erosions (see Fig. 9.9). This bone damage can be reversed by treating the cause of the excess PTH.

Renal osteodystrophy

Renal osteodystrophy is the collective term for all the skeletal changes occurring in chronic renal disease.

Pathology

Renal osteodystrophy is caused by:
- Inadequate renal tissue for making vitamin D—leads to osteomalacia.
- High serum phosphate—precipitates hyperparathyroidism.
- Prolonged haemodialysis—inhibits calcification of bone matrix and produces osteomalacia.
- Steroids—may induce osteoporosis or avascular necrosis.

Clinical features

The clinical features of renal osteodystrophy are similar to those of osteitis fibrosa cystica and osteomalacia. Osteosclerosis occurs and chronically there are metastatic calcifications in the skin, eyes, joints, and arterial walls.

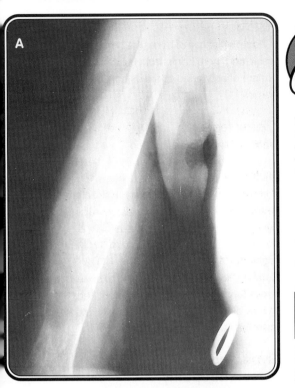

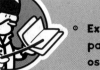

MISCELLANEOUS DISEASES OF BONE

Paget's disease of bone

Paget's disease of bone is also known as osteitis deformans. It is a disease of disordered bone formation and resorption. It commonly occurs in people over 40 years of age and affects males more than females. Paget's disease of bone usually occurs in White populations of the Western world; it is rare in Asians and Africans.

Classification

Paget's disease of bone affects either one bone (15%) or several (85%). Bones affected are the tibia, femur, ileum, vertebrae, humerus, and skull (Fig. 9.10).

Causes

The cause of Paget's disease of bone is unknown, but may be due to infection of osteoclasts by paramyxovirus, measles virus, or respiratory syncytial virus.

Pathology

Paget's disease of bone occurs in three phases. These are the:

- Initial osteolytic phase, when there is a huge increase in osteoclastic activity.
- Mixed osteoclast/osteoblast phase, when there is disordered activity and a mosaic pattern of bone is produced.
- Quiescent osteosclerotic phase, when new sclerotic bone is produced after a period of years.

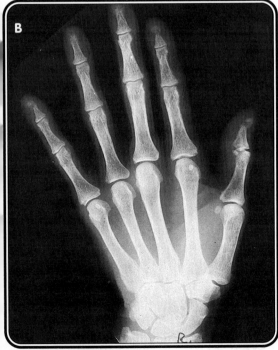

Fig. 9.9 Hyperparathyroidism. (A) Radiograph showing large destructive lesion (brown tumour) in the lower half of the humerus. (Courtesy of Dr P.G. Bullough.) (B) Radiograph showing subperiosteal erosion of the cortical surfaces of the phalanges. (Courtesy of Dr A. Norman.)

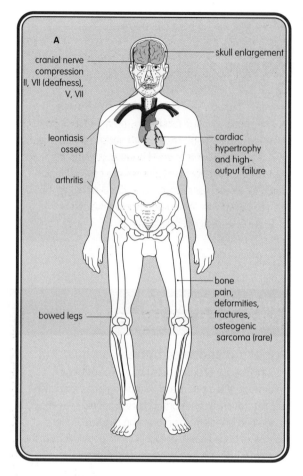

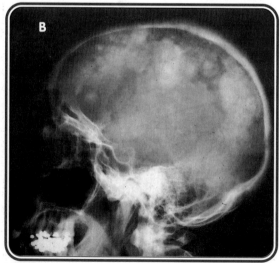

Fig. 9.10 Paget's disease of bone. (A) General features, and (B) radiograph of skull in late stage showing patchy sclerosis and loss of diploic architecture. (Courtesy of Dr P.G. Bullough.)

Histology

In Paget's disease of bone, the bone is thickened but weak, and there is intertrabecular fibrosis and a mosaic pattern of new bone as the osteoid is very bulky and porous.

Clinical features

Fractures and coarsened facial bones in Paget's disease of bone lead to a leonine facies, bone pain, and fractures. There may be deafness due to nerve compression by the overgrown skull. Serum alkaline phosphatase and calcium levels are raised and hydroxyproline is present in the urine.

Complications

Complications of Paget's disease of bone include secondary osteoarthritis, high-output heart failure due to new blood vessels forming shunts, and Paget's sarcoma (% of cases).

Hypertrophic pulmonary osteoarthropathy

Hypertrophic pulmonary osteoarthropathy is an uncommon, idiopathic condition causing changes to bones and joints.

Pathology

In hypertrophic pulmonary osteoarthropathy there is:
- New periosteal bone formation in the distal long bones, wrists, ankles, and proximal phalanges.
- Arthritis of adjacent joints.
- Clubbing of digits.

Clinical features

Hypertrophic pulmonary osteoarthropathy is associated with lung cancer or pleural mesothelioma, and there is usually an increased blood flow to the limbs. Resection of the tumours usually leads to regression of the condition.

- Describe the features of Paget's disease of bone.
- What does hypertrophic osteodystrophy lead to?

TUMOURS OF THE SKELETON

Metastatic tumours of the skeleton

Metastatic tumours of the skeleton are much more common than primary bone tumours, particularly in adults.

Metastases arising from the breast, lung, kidney, and thyroid are lytic, whereas those from the prostate are sclerotic.

Cartilage-forming tumours
Chondroma and endochondroma

Cartilage-forming tumours are benign tumours composed of mature hyaline cartilage. Those within bone are endochondromas, and those on the surface, subperiosteal chondromas (Fig. 9.11).

Epidemiology

Males are more likely to develop cartilage-forming tumours than females—usually between 20 and 50 years of age.

Types

There are two types of cartilage-forming tumours—solitary and multiple.

Multiple tumours involve non-familial types—endochromatosis or Ollier's disease—and familial types—Mafucci's syndrome. Familial types are associated with haemangiomas.

Clinical features

Features of cartilage-forming tumours include bone pain and fractures. The tumours consist of cartilage nests and arise at the epiphyses. There is a risk of chondrosarcoma in multiple lesions, especially if the condition is familial.

Chondrosarcoma

Chondrosarcomas are malignant tumours of cartilage. They grow slowly and occur half as frequently as osteosarcomas—75% are primary and the rest form endochondromas, osteochondromas, and chondroblastomas.

Epidemiology

Males are more likely to develop chondrosarcomas than are females—usually over 30 years of age.

Types

Chondrosarcomas are graded from 1 to 3 according to nuclear atypia. Five-year survival rates range from 90% (low grade) to 40% (high grade).

Clinical features

Radiographs of chondrosarcomas show localized areas of bone destruction mottled with dense calcified spots. High-grade tumours spread haematogeneously, notably to the lungs. Typical sites are central bones such as the pelvis, scapula, and ribs. Histology shows large, gelatinous, lobulated tumours that are translucent when cut and show necrosis and spotty calcifications.

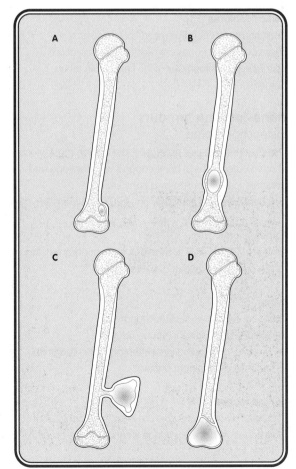

Fig. 9.11 Benign bone tumours. (A) osteoma, (B) endochondroma and chondroma, (C) osteochondroma, and (D) giant-cell tumour.

Chondroblastoma

Chondroblastomas, or Codman's tumours, are rare benign tumours that affect the epiphyses of young people. The tumours, which are composed of chondroblasts arranged in sheets, have a grooved nucleus and a surrounding calcified network; osteoclast-like cells may also be present.

Chondromyxoid fibroma

Chondromyxoid fibromas are rare benign tumours composed of cartilage matrix, and fibrous and myxoid tissue.

Epidemiology

Males are more likely to develop chondromyxoid fibromas than females—usually between 10 and 30 years of age.

Clinical features

Radiographs of chondromyxoid fibromas show circumscribed lucencies with scattered calcifications, usually in the metaphyses of the tibia, fibula, and humerus.

Bone-forming tumours

Osteochondroma

Osteochondromas, or exostoses, are benign mushroom-shaped outgrowths of bone capped with cartilage and attached to the skeleton by a bony stalk. Osteochondromas can grow up to 20 cm in diameter.

Epidemiology

Males are more likely to develop osteochondromas than females—usually under 20 years of age.

Types

There are two types of osteochondroma:
- Solitary, developing in young adults.
- Multiple, developing in children and inherited in an autosomal dominant pattern.

Clinical features

In osteochondroma, lesions are near the epiphyses of long bones. Malignant change is rare, but can occur in multiple lesions.

Osteoma

Osteomas are slow-growing benign tumours composed of sclerotic bone that is well formed (see Fig. 9.11). Osteomas are unlikely to become malignant.

Epidemiology

Both young and middle-aged people can develop osteomas.

Type

There are two types of osteoma. These are:
- Solitary, developing in middle age.
- Multiple, developing in young people and often associated with polyposis coli (Gardner's syndrome).

Clinical features

Osteomas are likely to protrude from cortical surfaces, especially the skull and facial bones. They are usually harmless unless the location compromises organ function, e.g. growth on the inner skull.

Osteoid osteoma and osteoblastoma

Osteoid osteomas are small benign tumours surrounded by a dense sclerotic ring of new bone, and are usually less than 2 cm in diameter.

Osteoblastomas (also called giant osteoid osteomas) have a similar histology, without the sclerotic ring, and are usually more than 2 cm in diameter.

Epidemiology

Males are more likely to develop osteoid osteomas and osteoblastomas than are females—usually between 5 and 25 years of age.

Clinical features

Osteoid osteomas are located in the cortex of the tibia and femur, and are very painful. Radiographs show a small radiolucent 'nest' of trabecular bone surrounded by a ring of dense sclerotic bone. The nest consists of osteoid, osteoblasts, and a vascular stroma.

Osteoblastomas are less painful than osteoid osteomas and are found in the vertebrae and long bones. They may become malignant and form osteosarcomas.

Osteosarcoma

Osteosarcomas are the most common type of primary

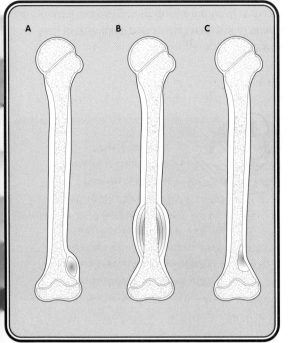

Fig. 9.12 Malignant bone tumours: (A) osteosarcoma, (B) Ewing's sarcoma, and (C) metastatic bone tumours.

bone tumour (Fig. 9.12). They are composed of osteocytes and osteoid. Osteosarcomas are thought to be related to the retinoblastoma and p53 genes. They grow quickly and, with combination therapy, have a 60% 5-year survival rate. Some histological variants, such as juxtacortical and periosteal types, have a better prognosis.

Epidemiology
Males are more likely to develop osteosarcomas than females—usually up to 20 years of age, although the elderly with pre-existing bone tumours are also at risk.

Clinical features
Osteosarcomas are found in the medullary cavity of metaphyses of long bones (especially near the knee) and, in the elderly, in flat bones. They produce bone pain, tenderness, and swelling. Osteosarcomas are usually a complication of Paget's disease of bone . Radiographs show elevated periosteum (Codman's triangle) due to new bone growth under the periosteum. There may be haematogenous spread to the lungs.

Fibrous and fibro-osseous tumours
Fibroma
Fibromas are benign, well-defined tumours composed of fibroblasts and collagenous tissue. They are usually found in the ovary, but may develop elsewhere.

Fibrous dysplasia
Fibrous dysplasia is a benign disorder in which there is progressive replacement of bone. This takes place by fibroblasts that are arranged in a regular pattern with small spicules of immature bone. As a result, the bones become structurally weakened.

Epidemiology
Fibrous dysplasia affects children and young adults.

Types
There are three types of fibrous dysplasia. These are:
- Monostotic (70%).
- Polyostotic (25%).
- Polyostotic and associated with endocrinopathies (5%).

Albright's syndrome is fibrous dysplasia with precocious sexual development and irregular skin pigmentation.

Clinical features
Fibrous dysplasia is found in the ribs, femur, tibia, and skull. There is a 'ground glass' appearance on radiographs and *café-au-lait* spots over affected bones. Rarely, some can become osteosarcomas.

Miscellaneous tumours
Ewing's sarcoma
Ewing's sarcomas are aggressive malignant tumours of primitive neural differentiation (see Fig. 9.12). These grey tumours contain small round cells growing in sheets around blood vessels, and show focal necrosis and haemorrhage. However, they respond to drugs and have an overall five-year survival of 60%.

Epidemiology
Females are more likely to develop Ewing's sarcoma than males—usually under 25 years of age. Ewing's sarcoma is very rare in Black children.

Clinical features

Ewing's sarcoma presents as a soft tissue mass—periosteal 'onion-skinning' is seen on radiographs.

Giant-cell tumour

Giant-cell tumours, or osteoclastomas, are low-grade malignant tumours of giant multinucleate cells and stroma; 10% form metastases (see Fig. 9.11).

Epidemiology

Females are more likely to develop giant-cell tumours than males—usually between 20 and 40 years of age.

Clinical features

Radiographs of giant cell tumours show large lytic 'soap-bubble' lesions with absent calcified spots. These can often be mistaken for 'brown tumours' that occur in hyperparathyroidism. Giant-cell tumours are found at the metaphyses and epiphyses of long bones, especially the knees.

- **Describe the differences between metastatic and primary tumours in the skeleton.**
- **Give a simple classification of tumours of the skeleton.**
- **Distinguish between benign and malignant tumours.**

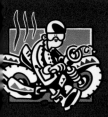

10. Pathology of the Joints and Connective Tissues

Degenerative arthropathy
Osteoarthritis
Epidemiology

Osteoarthritis is the most common type of arthritis. It affects more than 20% of the population of the United Kingdom, and has a male:female ratio of 1:2.

Osteoarthritis is particularly common in the elderly and, although it occurs worldwide, is less common in Black people.

Aetiology

Osteoarthritis can be either primary or secondary.

Osteoarthritis arising from no obvious cause is known as primary osteoarthritis. Predisposing factors include age (it is most common in the elderly), genetic factors, biomechanical factors (e.g. lifestyle), and systemic factors such as obesity.

Secondary osteoarthritis is less common than primary osteoarthritis and tends to affect younger people. Causes include congenital abnormalities, trauma, occupational hazards (e.g. the knee joint in footballers), avascular necrosis (e.g. sickle-cell disease), and other associated arthropathies or bone diseases.

Pathology

Osteoarthritis most commonly affects weightbearing joints such as the hip and knee. Other sites also affected are the vertebrae, hands, and feet.

In the early stages of osteoarthritis there is degeneration of cartilage (Fig. 10.1). This involves:
- The breakdown of cartilage due to the release of enzymes from chondrocytes—the stimulus for this is unknown.
- The swelling and splitting of cartilage due to the uptake of water. The loss of cartilage is variable, ranging from irregularity of the surface to full-thickness loss.
- The inflammation of synovium and joint capsule due to debris from the cartilage.

In the later stages, there are secondary changes in bone as a consequence of degeneration. This involves:
- Articulation of bone with bone, resulting in thickening and polishing (eburnation) of subarticular bone.
- Development of cysts in subarticular bone.
- Formation of osteophytes at articular margins.
- Hyperplasia of synovium due to inflammation.
- Immobility of a joint, resulting in disuse atrophy of muscle.

Clinical features

Osteoarthritis usually presents at 50 years of age, although secondary osteoarthritis presents earlier.
Symptoms include:
- Intermittent or chronic pain at affected sites, which is worse upon exertion.
- Joint stiffness following rest, e.g. early morning stiffness, which improves after a little activity.

Signs include:
- Swelling at affected joints due to effusions and osteophyte formation.
- Joint deformities with crepitus upon movement.
- Muscular wasting due to limited use of a joint.

In the hands, the presence of Heberden's nodes [swellings at the distal interphalangeal joints (DIP)] and Bouchard's nodes [swellings at the proximal interphalangeal joints (PIP)] should be sought.

Joints are usually affected bilaterally and symmetrically, although a unilateral pattern may be seen.

Diagnosis

Osteoarthritis is diagnosed clinically from the pattern of joints involved and the absence of systemic features.

A plain X-ray demonstrates narrowing of the joint space, and the presence of osteophytes, subchondral cysts, and osteosclerosis.

Blood tests are negative for rheumatoid factor and antinuclear antibodies (ANAs). The erythrocyte sedimentation rate (ESR) is normal and there is no evidence of anaemia or abnormality of calcium metabolism.

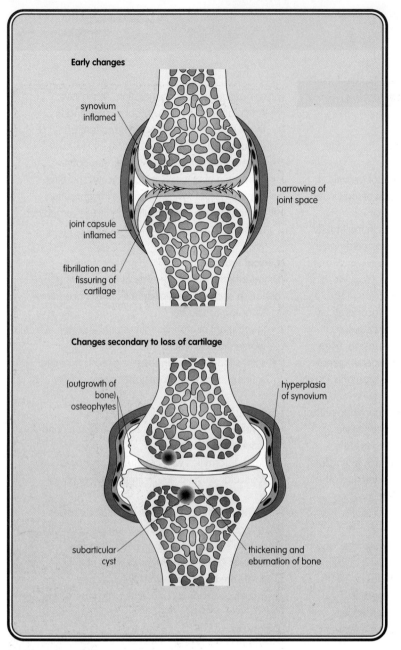

Fig. 10.1 Pathological changes in osteoarthritis. Early changes and changes secondary to loss of cartilage.

Early changes

synovium inflamed

narrowing of joint space

joint capsule inflamed

fibrillation and fissuring of cartilage

Changes secondary to loss of cartilage

(outgrowth of bone) osteophytes

hyperplasia of synovium

subarticular cyst

thickening and eburnation of bone

Analysis of synovial fluid shows an increase in volume and the presence of white blood cells and crystals. Culture is negative.

Complications
Osteoarthritis has the potential to cause disability because of decreased mobility.

Management
Osteoarthritis is treated by non-steroidal anti-inflammatory drugs (NSAIDs) and analgesics to control pain, a balance between exercise and rest, and advising the patient on the progressive nature of the disease. Weight loss should be discussed if appropriate.

Surgery may be needed to replace severely diseased joints.

Prognosis

Osteoarthritis is a progressive disease—affected joints slowly get worse and other joints also become involved.

Inflammatory arthropathies

Rheumatoid arthritis: adult form

Epidemiology

Rheumatoid arthritis is a common multisystemic disease affecting at least 1% of Caucasians; the male:female ratio is 1:3.

Aetiology

The cause of rheumatoid arthritis is unknown, although it is believed to involve an initiating factor that results in complex immunological changes. There are a number of possible hypotheses.

Evidence supporting autoimmune mechanisms in rheumatoid arthritis include:

- The presence of rheumatoid factor (an autoantibody).
- Circulating immune complexes—these are believed to be responsible for the extra-articular features.
- Defective T cell-mediated immunity.
- The presence of other autoimmune diseases.

Genetic factors are due to an association between Human leukocyte antigen (HLA) DR4 and DR1.

The initiating factor in rheumatoid arthritis has not been determined although possible candidates include the Epstein–Barr virus and parvoviruses.

Pathology

The most common sites affected in rheumatoid arthritis are the small joints of the hands (i.e. the PIP joints as opposed to the DIP joints in osteoarthritis). Other joints that may be involved include the wrist, elbow, shoulder, cervical spine, hip, and knee.

The inflammation associated with osteoarthritis is secondary to degeneration.

The disease process can be split into three stages (Fig. 10.2). These include:

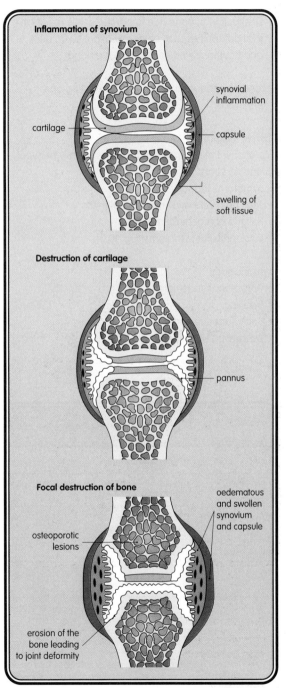

Fig. 10.2 Pathological changes in rheumatoid arthritis. Inflammation of synovium, destruction of cartilage, and focal destruction of bone.

- Inflammation of the synovium—there is an infiltration of lymphocytes and macrophages.
- Destruction of cartilage—pannus (a layer of chronically inflamed fibrous tissue) extends across the cartilage, destroying it.
- Destruction of bone due to pannus—this results in joint deformities (e.g. ulnar deviation, swan neck, and boutonnière deformities in the hand).

Secondary changes include muscle wasting and osteoporosis.

Clinical features
Age of onset of rheumatoid arthritis is usually between 35 and 45 years.

Symptoms include:
- Joint pain with early morning stiffness.
- Fatigue and general malaise.
- Extra-articular symptoms (Fig. 10.3).

Signs include:
- Warm and tender joints.
- Swelling.
- Subcutaneous nodules.
- Decreased movement.

In the later stages the joint deformities mentioned above and muscle wasting may be seen.
Splenomegaly and lymphadenopathy may be present.

The joints are affected symmetrically and the disease is progressive with remissions.

Diagnosis
The diagnosis of rheumatoid arthritis is clinically from the pattern of joints involved, the presence of rheumatoid nodules, and episodes of remission.

About 80% of patients show the presence of rheumatoid factor and 30% ANAs. The ESR and C-reactive protein levels are raised. There is an associated anaemia and thrombocytosis.

A plain X-ray will demonstrate narrowing of joint space with the presence of subchondral cysts. In addition there may be osteoporosis in bone adjacent to the affected joint and focal erosions of bone.

Synovial fluid is usually turbid and green/yellow in colour. White blood cells are present and culture is negative.

Complications
Rheumatoid arthritis can cause secondary osteoarthritis and/or septic arthritis.

Rheumatoid arthritis can also cause be disabling.

Extra-articular features of rheumatoid disease	
Site	**Manifestation**
nerves	carpal tunnel syndrome, peripheral neuropathy ('glove and stocking' sensory loss)
skin	subcutaneous nodules (particularly on extensor aspect of forearm near elbow), vasculitic lesions
blood vessels	vasculitis
eyes	episcleritis, scleritis, secondary Sjögren's syndrome (i.e. triad of dry mouth, dry eyes, and arthritis)
chest	intrapulmonary nodules, pleural effusions, fibrosing alveolitis, Caplan's syndrome
heart	myocarditis, pericarditis, pericardial effusion
kidney	amyloidosis, impaired renal function may be side effect of drug treatment
soft tissues around joints	bursitis, tenosynovitis

Fig. 10.3 Extra-articular features of rheumatoid disease.

Management
Rheumatoid arthritis is treated by NSAIDs to control the pain, and immunosuppressive drugs such as penicillamine, gold, and corticosteroids. Side effects of treatment include gastrointestinal bleeding and renal impairment.

Treatment is aimed at the complications.

Prognosis
The progression of rheumatoid arthritis is variable with more joints becoming involved.

Rheumatoid arthritis: juvenile form
The juvenile form of rheumatoid arthritis occurs before the age of 16 years; the prognosis is worse than in adults.

Seronegative arthritides
The seronegative arthritides are a group of related disorders. They are similar because they:

- Are often associated with HLA B27 (human leucocyte antigen B27).
- Are negative for rheumatoid factor and other autoantibodies.
- Have a familial tendency.
- Are more common in White people.

Patients may present with several different disorders, occurring either simultaneously or at different times.

Ankylosing spondylitis
Epidemiology
Ankylosing spondylitis is the most common cause of inflammatory back pain in young adults (Fig. 10.4).

The symptomatic disorder is more common in males although the incidence in both sexes has been suggested as equal, with women showing milder symptoms.

Aetiology
There is a familial tendency in ankylosing spondylitis, with the HLA B27 association occurring in 90% of affected individuals.

Pathology
The spinal joints are affected in ankylosing spondylitis. Inflammation starts in the lumbar spine and sacro-iliac joints and extends proximally. The inflammation starts at sites of ligamentous insertions (enthesis), resulting in enthesiopathy.

Initially there is inflammation of the ligaments around the vertebrae.

Healing involves fibrosis and ossification of the ligaments. Fusion may occur and the spine becomes inflexible and rigid ('bamboo spine').

Clinical features
Most patients with ankylosing spondylitis present in their late teens or early adulthood.

Symptoms include:
- Back pain, pelvic pain, and joint pain in the lower limbs.
- Systemic manifestations, including iritis and aortic valve incompetence.

Signs that may be present include:
- Kyphosis.
- Limited spinal flexion.
- Decreased chest expansion.

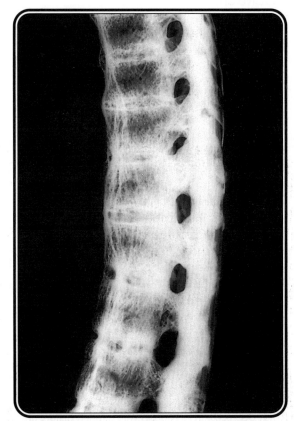

Fig. 10.4 Radiograph of a sagittal section through the vertebral column showing ankylosing spondylitis. There is complete fusion of the spine and apophyseal joints, and across the intervertebral disc. (Courtesy of Dr P.G. Bullough.)

Diagnosis
Ankylosing spondylitis is diagnosed by the presence of HLA B27 (90%), although unaffected individuals may also carry this antigen (16%).

ESR and C-reactive protein levels are often raised.

A spinal radiograph may demonstrate calcification and ossification, the so-called tramline appearance.

Management
Ankylosing spondylitis is usually treated with NSAIDs, immunosuppressive drugs such as sulphasalazine, regular exercise to maintain movement, and hip replacement (occasionally required if the hip is ankylosed).

Prognosis
Although ankylosing spondylitis is progressive, most patients are able to lead a normal life.

Reactive arthritis
There are two types of reactive arthritis. These occur after:
- Genital infection with *Chlamydia*.
- Gastrointestinal infection with *Salmonella*, *Campylobacter*, or *Shigella*.

Reactive arthritis is more common in males and is the most common cause of arthritis in young males.

About 80% of patients show an association with HLA B27, suggesting an autoimmune process.

An example of reactive arthritis is Reiter's syndrome, i.e.:
- A triad of arthritis, urethritis/cervicitis, and conjunctivitis. The arthritis usually affects the knees or ankles (asymmetrical oligoarthritis), although axial disease may occur.
- The changes seen histologically are similar to those of rheumatoid arthritis.
- Diagnosis is clinical.
- Although symptoms may clear spontaneously, a large number of patients will suffer recurrences. In a minority, severe spondylitis may develop.

Psoriatic arthritis
Psoriatic arthritis occurs in 5–10% of psoriasis sufferers. It may also occur in individuals with a family history of psoriasis.

HLA B27 association is often seen if spondylitis is also present.

The DIP joints are most affected; axial involvement may also occur. The joint changes are similar to those of rheumatoid arthritis.

The diagnosis is clinical, although an X-ray may show erosions and periarticular osteoporosis.

Treatment is with NSAIDs and analgesics. Immunosuppressive drugs may also be used. In a minority of cases, severe destruction of bone may occur, i.e. 'arthritis mutilans'.

Arthritis associated with gastrointestinal disease
Arthritis can be associated with gastrointestinal conditions such as Crohn's disease or ulcerative colitis.

The sites affected are the knees, ankles, and elbows.

Other non-articular symptoms of inflammatory bowel disease may be present, e.g. erythema nodosum.

The severity of the arthritis reflects the activity of the inflammatory bowel disease. Most episodes resolve within a few months.

Arthritis associated with systemic disease
Behçet's syndrome
Behçet's syndrome is a rare condition of unknown aetiology. The main features are polyarthritis, iritis, and oral/genital ulceration. Less commonly there may be neurological, skin, or gastrointestinal symptoms.

Oral steroids are used to treat Behçet's syndrome.

Still's disease
Still's disease is the most common cause of chronic juvenile arthritis, i.e. arthritis occurring in a person under 16 years of age.

Some forms of Still's disease are similar to rheumatoid arthritis.

Systemic symptoms include a salmon-coloured rash, spiking fever, lymphadenopathy, splenomegaly, and pericarditis.

The number of joints affected is variable, depending on the subtype of Still's disease.

Most patients recover spontaneously before early adulthood.

Sarcoidosis
Sarcoidosis usually occurs in association with erythema nodosum although a transient polyarthritis or an acute monoarthritis may also occur.

Neuropathic joint disease (Charcot's joint)

In neuropathic joint disease, or Charcot's joint, loss of sensation results in traumatic joint damage.

The conditions associated with Charcot's joint are:
- Diabetes mellitus, where joints in the feet are affected.
- Tabes dorsalis following syphilis, where the ankle and knee joints are affected.
- Leprosy, where the joint affected varies according to the site of sensory loss.

Haemodialysis

Arthritis can arise as a result of haemodialysis, due to the deposition of amyloid in the joints and pericortical tissues. Oxilate crystal deposition may occur in chronic renal disorders.

Systemic lupus erythematosus

Systemic lupus erythematosus (SLE) is a connective tissue disorder usually presenting with joint symptoms resembling rheumatoid arthritis.

Crystal arthropathies
Definition

The crystal arthropathies are a group of disorders in which the deposition of crystals in joints leads to inflammation.

Gout
Epidemiology

Gout is more common in men, although some postmenopausal women may be affected.

Aetiology

In gout, hyperuricaemia results in the deposition of monosodium urate crystals in the joint.

In primary gout, the causes of hyperuricaemia are commonly idiopathic, usually due to impaired excretion. There is a familial tendency.

Secondary gout may occur as a result of:
- Increased production of uric acid, e.g. increased cell turnover in carcinomas and leukaemia, following chemotherapy, and in enzyme defects.
- Impaired excretion, e.g. renal failure, alcohol consumption, hyperlipidaemia, and diuretics.
- High purine intake in the diet.

Pathology

Uric acid is a product of DNA (purine) breakdown and is normally excreted in the urine.

Excess uric acid results in the deposition of crystals in:
- Joints—the most commonly affected being the metatarsophalangeal (MTP) joint in the big toe. The ankle joint may also be affected.
- Soft tissues—this may lead to the formation of tophi (palpable masses).
- The urinary tract, in the form of urate stones.

The deposition of crystals in the synovium and periarticular soft tissues causes an acute inflammatory reaction. This may be precipitated by alcohol, diet, surgery, or drugs.

Chronic gouty arthritis occurs following recurrent attacks. This is characterized by cartilage degeneration, synovial hyperplasia, and secondary osteoarthritis.

Clinical

Patients with gout present between the ages of 20 and 60 years, although most commonly in middle age.

An acute attack involves an extremely painful monoarthritis of sudden onset. The affected joint is oedematous and red; more than one joint may be affected in certain cases.

Diagnosis

The presence of tophi on the earlobes or around joints may aid in the diagnosis of gout.

Synovial fluid demonstrates the presence of needle-shaped crystals, which are diagnostic These crystals are negatively birefringent. Neutrophils are also found.

Plasma uric acid levels are raised at >0.5 mmol/L, and there is also a raised ESR and white cell count.

Management

An acute attack of gout is treated with NSAIDs and aspiration of joint effusions.

Allopurinol, a drug that decreases uric acid synthesis, is used long term. The patient should be advised to maintain a good fluid intake and avoid precipitating factors.

Complications

Renal disease is a complication of gout.

Hyperuricaemia is genetically associated with an increased risk of hypertension and coronary artery disease.

Prognosis

Attacks of gout may be infrequent, and treatment can reduce the extent of joint damage. However, renal complications are frequent.

Pseudogout

Pseudogout is a condition that may mimic gout. It is more common in the elderly.

In pseudogout, calcium pyrophosphate crystals are deposited in the articular cartilage. Inflammation results if the crystals are shed into the joint space.

When pseudogout occurs in people younger than 60 years of age, it is often associated with hyperparathyroidism and haemochromatosis.

The joints most commonly affected are the knee, wrist, shoulder, and ankle.

Pseudogout can be differentiated from gout by the presence of brick-shaped crystals in the synovial fluid which are positively birefringent.

Infectious (septic) arthritis
Epidemiology

Infectious (septic) arthritis is an uncommon condition, usually affecting children and young adults.

Aetiology

Infectious arthritis is usually caused by bacteria such as *Staphylococcus aureus*, *Streptococcus pyogenes*, *Neisseria gonorrhoea,* and *Haemophilus influenzae,* and Gram-negative organisms. Tuberculous arthritis is now rare.

There are several predisposing factors. These include:

- Prosthetic joints.
- Drug addiction.
- Age between 5 and 15 years.
- Diabetes mellitus.
- Immunosuppressive drugs.
- Rheumatoid arthritis.

A viral cause, such as rubella or mumps, is less common.

Pathology

In infectious arthritis the infecting organism gains access to the joint:

- Haematogeneously.
- As a result of local trauma.
- By direct spread from adjacent foci of infection.

Clinical

Only one joint is usually affected in infectious arthritis, the patient presenting with a painful, swollen, and erythematous joint and associated fever.

Diagnosis

Synovial fluid is turbid in infectious arthritis, and white blood cells are present. Culture is positive. Patients need an X-ray to exclude trauma.

Management

Intravenous antibiotic treatment should be started immediately infectious arthritis is diagnosed. This is initially 'blind' until the culture results are available. Treatment with oral antibiotics is continued for 6 weeks.

Drainage of the joint is needed to remove debris. The joint should also be immobilized.

Prognosis

Infectious arthritis can be life threatening, hence the importance of immediate treatment.

Recovery can take from a few days to a few weeks.

- Give a simple classification of the arthropathies.
- Describe osteoarthritis, rheumatoid arthritis, and gout.

DISORDERS AFFECTING SPECIFIC JOINTS

Disorders of the back
Congenital abnormalities

Lumbarization and sacralization are inconsequential anatomical anomalies. Lumbarization is when S1 remains as a vertebra, and sacralization is fusion of the body of L5 with the sacrum.

Hemivertebrae are formed on one lateral side only (Fig. 10.5). The body is wedge-shaped, causing the spine to angle laterally at this site.

Torticollis

Torticollis is a contracted sternocleidomastoid muscle on one side of the body only. It is caused by poor blood supply during a birth injury. The head is tilted and rotated to one side and there is facial asymmetry (Fig. 10.6).

Management

Torticollis is corrected by surgery.

Scoliosis

Scoliosis is the lateral curvature of the spine (Fig. 10.7). The deformity may be mobile (reversible) or fixed (permanent).

Mobile scoliosis may be postural, compensatory (to a short leg or pelvic tilt), or sciatic (with disc prolapse and muscle spasm).

Aetiology

Fixed scoliosis can be caused by:
- Congenital vertebral abnormalities.
- Hemivertebrae.
- Asymmetrical muscle weakness.
- Muscular dystrophies.

Fixed scoliosis may be idiopathic in infants and adolescents.

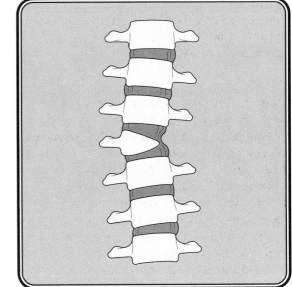

Fig. 10.5 Hemivertebra in the spine, producing scoliosis.

Management

Fixed scoliosis can be treated either conservatively with exercise or by wearing supportive splints, or surgically.

Kyphosis

Kyphosis is excessive posterior curvature of the spine that is either gently rounded or sharply angled (Fig. 10.8). It can be a progressive deformity.

Fig. 10.6 Features of torticollis. (Courtesy of Dr G.D. Perkin.)

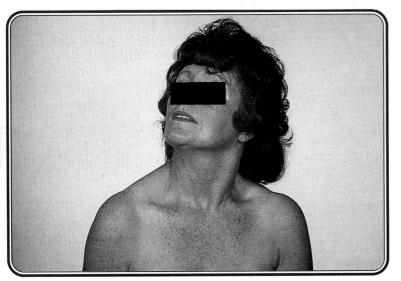

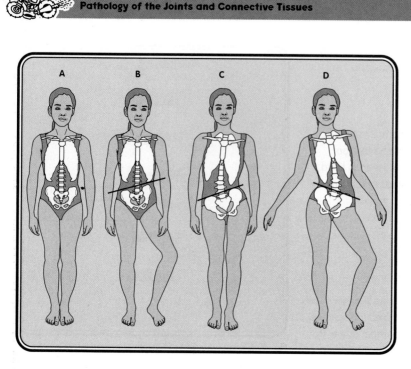

Fig. 10.7 Types of scoliosis. (A) Normal posture, and scoliosis due to (B) sciatica, (C) short leg, and (D) fixed deformity.

Kyphosis can be caused by tuberculosis of the spine, fractured vertebrae, ankylosing spondylitis, and spinal tumours.

Lordosis

Lordosis is excessive anterior curvature of the spine, usually in the lumbar region (see Fig. 10.8). It may be due to bad posture or compensatory for hip deformities.

Disc prolapse

Disc prolapse usually occurs in the lumbar region—the nucleus pulposus herniates through a weak part of the annulus fibrosus (Fig. 10.9).

Sudden pain can be felt in the lumbar region (lumbago) or, if there is compression of a nerve root, may radiate to the buttocks and legs (sciatica). There is limited flexion and extension.

Management

Disc prolapse should be treated with analgesics, by injection of chymopapain (dissolves protruding disc), or disc excision.

Spondylolisthesis

In spondylolisthesis there is forward displacement of a lumbar vertebral body on to the one below. There may be pain and a 'step' can be palpated over the spine.

Management

Spondylolisthesis can be treated conservatively by wearing a corset, or surgically by fusion of the vertebral joints.

Spinal stenosis

Spinal stenosis is narrowing of the spinal canal. It may be caused by long-term osteoarthritis and disc degeneration.

Standing and walking lead to severe pain in the buttocks and thighs, as nerves and blood vessels are cramped. The pain is relieved by rest.

Management

Spinal stenosis is treated by the removal of osteophytes and part of the bony canal.

Back strain

Without an adequate warm-up, the muscles and ligaments of the lumbar spine can be strained during unaccustomed or sudden movements.

Management

Back strain is treated by rest, analgesics, application of heat, and gradual mobilization.

Tuberculosis in the back

Tuberculosis (TB) of the spine is called Pott's disease (Fig. 10.10). The spine is the most likely part of the skeleton to be affected by TB.

In Pott's disease, the vertebral bodies collapse onto each other, creating a sharply angled 'gibbus' deformity. There is also a risk of cord compression (Pott's paraplegia), chronic discharging sinus, and the spread of TB to other organs.

Management

Pott's disease is treated with antituberculous drugs. The pus is drained, any dead bone removed, and the vertebrae fused.

Arthritic disease in the back

Osteoarthritis

Osteoarthritis in the back tends to affect the thoracic or lumbar vertebrae (Fig. 10.11). It usually occurs in people who lift heavy objects or those with previous injuries, such as disc prolapse or degeneration. There is narrowing of the intervertebral discs and osteophyte formation in the lateral joint margins; these predispose to spinal stenosis and spondylolisthesis.

Rheumatoid arthritis

When rheumatoid arthritis occurs in the back, it often

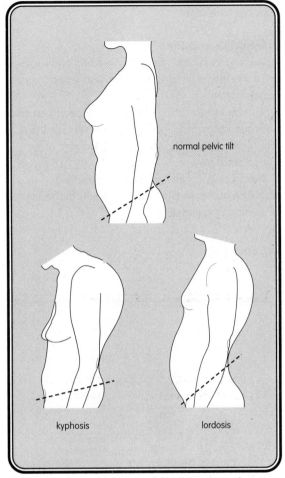

Fig. 10.8 Features of kyphosis and lordosis. Normal posture, kyphosis, and lordosis.

Fig. 10.9 Intervertebral disc prolapse.

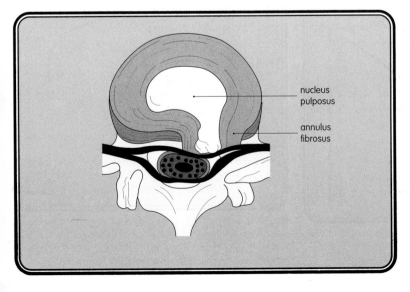

affects the cervical vertebrae. There is diffuse pain and impaired movement.

Ankylosing spondylitis

Ankylosing spondylitis affects the vertebral and sacro-iliac joints before progressing to the limb joints. It occurs mostly in men.

There is erosion of the normal articular cartilage and underlying bone, then replacement with fibrous tissue, which also ossifies. This causes derangement of the normal structures.

Diffuse pain, a stiffened spine, and marked restriction of chest expansion are the principal features of ankylosing spondylitis.

Pain referred to the back

Retroperitoneal disease in the abdomen (duodenal ulcer, pancreatic cancer, aneurysm) may give back pain.

Period pain and sciatic pain also radiate to the back.

Shoulder joint
Dislocation of the shoulder joint

A dislocated shoulder joint is a very common injury, usually caused by falling on to an outstretched arm, e.g. when playing rugby. The joint may be displaced in different directions, but anterior displacement of the humeral head to below the coracoid process is the most common occurrence.

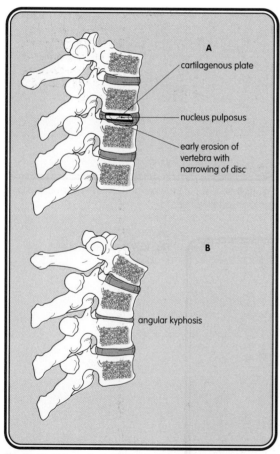

Fig. 10.10 Tuberculosis (Pott's disease) of the spine showing (A) erosion of vertebra and (B) subsequent collapse in front, resulting in angular curvature.

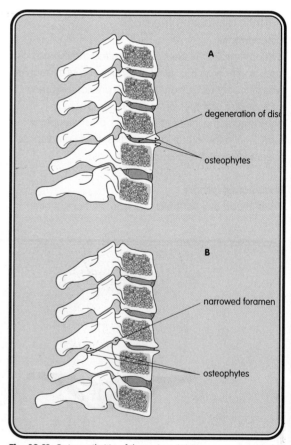

Fig. 10.11 Osteoarthritis of the spine. (A) Degeneration and narrowing of intervertebral disc forming osteophytes anteriorly. (B) Articular cartilage is worn away and marginal osteophytes surround the intervertebral foramen.

Complications

Complications of a dislocated shoulder include neural (circumflex axillary nerve) and arterial (axillary artery) damage, joint stiffness, and recurrent dislocations.

Management

A dislocated shoulder is treated by reducing the joint and immobilizing it for about 3 weeks.

Painful arc syndrome

In painful arc syndrome, shoulder abduction causes pain in the mid-ranges but not extremes of movement, i.e. between 45 and 150 degrees. Degeneration is the underlying defect and pain is due to impingement of an inflamed structure between the greater tuberosity and the acromion (Fig. 10.12).

Aetiology

Painful arc syndrome is caused by incomplete tearing of the supraspinatus tendon, supraspinatus tendonitis, subacromial bursitis, and fracture of the greater tuberosity of the humerus.

The lesions may be associated with supraspinatus tendon calcification (perhaps a variation of crystal arthropathy), rheumatoid arthritis, or acromioclavicular joint osteoarthritis.

Management

Painful arc syndrome is treated with hydrocortisone injections and surgery.

Rotator cuff tears

Rotator cuff tears are partial tears that often occur

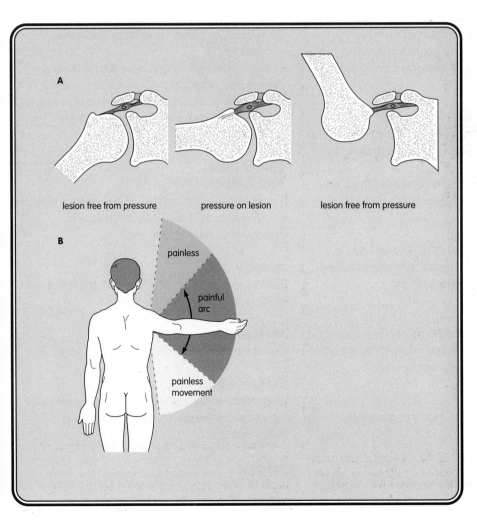

Fig. 10.12
Mechanism and aetiology of painful arc syndrome: (A) mechanical basis, and (B) areas of pain.

lesion free from pressure   pressure on lesion   lesion free from pressure

painless

painful arc

painless movement

with supraspinatus tendonitis, leading to painful arc syndromes. Complete tears limit shoulder abduction, cause joint pain at the shoulder tip and upper arm, and tenderness under the acromion. The tears are usually in the supraspinatus tendon (although subscapularis and infraspinatus may be involved) and allow communication between the joint capsule and the subacromial bursa, seen by arthroscopy.

Aetiology
Rotator cuff tears may be caused by age-related degeneration or a fall, e.g. in epileptic subjects.

Management
Rotator cuff tears are treated by repairing the tendon; this is better in young people with less degeneration.

Adhesive capsulitis (frozen shoulder)
Adhesive capsulitis or 'frozen shoulder' is a common but poorly understood condition affecting the glenohumeral joint. It causes pain and limitation of all movements (to about half the normal range) but no changes are seen on X-ray.

Aetiology and recovery
Adhesive capsulitis may follow a minor injury or be due to an autoimmune response to localized rotator cuff tissues.

Recovery follows the course of pain, stiffness, then recuperant phases. It may take months to heal.

Management
Adhesive capsulitis is treated initially with NSAIDs, analgesics, and gentle exercise. Joint manipulation is undertaken when the joint is stronger.

Biceps rupture
In biceps rupture, an aching in the shoulder often occurs after 'something snaps' during lifting. A 'ball' appears in the muscle belly on elbow flexion.

Aetiology
Biceps rupture may be caused by degenerative changes or a fall.

Management
As the function of the biceps remains intact during rupture, no treatment is required.

Biceps tendonitis
Biceps tendonitis is an uncommon condition, but rotator cuff tears may involve the long head of biceps, giving pain in the anterior shoulder. This is made worse on forced muscle contraction.

Management
Biceps tendonitis is treated by hydrocortisone injection.

Rheumatoid arthritis and osteoarthritis in the shoulder
Rheumatoid arthritis and osteoarthritis are not as common in the shoulder as they are in weightbearing hip and knee joints. Pain and restricted movement are treated by joint replacement.

Pain referred to the shoulder
Pain referred to the shoulder may occur via C5 to the deltoid, C6, C7, and C8 to the superior border of the scapula, or C3 from the diaphragm to the shoulder tip.

The brachial plexus and roots (e.g. prolapsed cervical disc, herpes zoster, cervical rib), upper arm, abdomen (e.g. cholecystitis, subphrenic abscess), and thorax (e.g. angina, pleurisy) may contribute to referred pain.

Elbow joint
Tennis elbow
Tennis elbow is inflammation of the common extensor attachment at the lateral epicondyle (lateral epicondylitis), causing pain.

Aetiology
Tennis elbow may be caused by hitting a tennis ball awkwardly during a backhand stroke.

Management
Tennis elbow is treated with steroid injections.

Golfer's elbow
Golfer's elbow is inflammation of the common flexor attachment at the medial epicondyle (medial epicondylitis).

Aetiology
Golfer's elbow may occur when a golfer hits the ground rather than the golfball.

Management
Golfer's elbow is treated with steroid injections.

Olecranon bursitis
Olecranon bursitis occurs after trauma, sepsis, rheumatoid arthritis, and gout. It involves a hot, painful swelling behind the olecranon.

Traumatic bursitis used to be called 'student's elbow'—caused by propping of the elbows on books for long periods.

Cubitus valgus and cubitus varus
Cubitus valgus is when the 'carrying angle' of the elbow joint is greater than the normal 10 degrees in men and 15 degrees in women (Fig. 10.13). It is caused by malunion of a previous lateral condylar fracture or retarded lateral epiphyseal growth. There may be an association with Turner's syndrome. Complications include ulnar neuritis and osteoarthritis.

Cubitus varus is the opposite deformity, with a decreased carrying angle (see Fig. 10.13). Its most common cause is malunion of a supracondylar fracture.

Management
Both cubitus valgus and cubitus varus may be corrected by osteotomy.

Ulnar neuritis
The ulnar nerve may be subjected to constriction (osteoarthritis, rheumatoid arthritis) or constant friction (cubitus valgus), as it lies in a groove behind the medial epicondyle. This can lead to nerve fibrosis and eventual ulnar neuropathy.

Complications
In ulnar neuritis there is hand clumsiness, reduced sensation over the little finger and the medial side of the ring finger, and weakened small muscles of the hand innervated by the nerve.

Management
Treatment of ulnar neuritis involves surgery for nerve release and transposition to the front of the elbow.

Loose bodies in the elbow joint
Loose bodies in the elbow joint may arise from

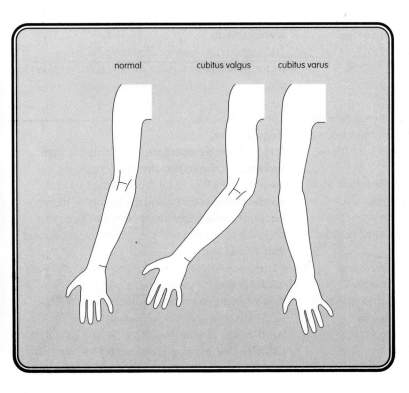

Fig. 10.13 Normal angle of the elbow, cubitus valgus, and cubitus varus.

osteochondral fractures, osteophytes of osteoarthritis, and other conditions such as synovial chondromatosis and osteochondritis dissecans.

Complications

Loose bodies in the elbow joint cause locking of the elbow. This occurs because the bodies become stuck between the bones, causing sharp pain and swelling.

Management

Loose bodies are treated by surgical removal.

Rheumatoid arthritis of the elbow

The elbow joint is involved in over half of all patients with rheumatoid arthritis. There is pain and limitation of movement in both the elbow and superior radiohumeral joints.

Management

Rheumatoid arthritis of the elbow is treated conservatively. Removal of the synovium or joint replacement may also be considered.

Wrist and hand joints

Osteoarthritis of the wrist and hand

The joints of the hand are commonly affected by osteoarthritis. The carpometacarpal joint of the thumb feels tender and there is limited abduction.

Aetiology

In osteoarthritis of the wrist and hand, the interphalangeal joints become painful and stiff, with osteophytes creating swellings; these are called Heberden's nodes at the DIP and Bouchard's nodes at the PIP joints.

The wrists are usually affected at a later stage after trauma (lower radius or scaphoid fracture).

Rheumatoid arthritis of the wrist and hand

Complications

The wrists and hands usually suffer a major loss of function and deformities in rheumatoid arthritis. Progressively there is synovitis of the proximal joints and tendon sheaths, then erosions, and finally joint derangement and tendon rupture leading to structural and functional loss.

The fingers have 'swan-neck' (hyperextended PIP joint and flexed DIP joint) or 'boutonnière' (flexed PIP joint, hyperextended DIP joint, and extended metacarpophalangeal joint) deformities (Fig. 10.14).

The thumb acquires a Z deformity. The MCP joints and wrists undergo subluxation so that the fingers show ulnar deviation.

The ulnar styloid and radial head become prominent. There may also be firm rheumatoid nodules on the extensor surfaces and the flexor tendons.

Management

Treatment for rheumatoid arthritis of the wrist and hand is complex and depends on the stage of disease progression.

De Quervain's tenosynovitis

De Quervain's tenosynovitis is inflammation of the fibrous sheath containing tendons of extensor pollicis brevis and abductor pollicis longus as it passes over the styloid process of the radius. Pain is felt at the styloid process of the radius, and there is tendon swelling and a palpable nodule proximal to the wrist joint on the radial aspect.

Aetiology

De Quervain's tenosynovitis may be caused by overuse of the tendons, e.g. wringing out washing.

Management

Treatment of De Quervain's tenosynovitis is by hydrocortisone injection or surgically splitting the tendon sheath.

Tendon lesions

'Trigger finger'

'Trigger finger' or digital stenosing synovitis is thickening of the tendon sheaths, constricting the flexor tendons (Fig. 10.15). It affects the ring and middle fingers in adults and the thumb in children. Extension of the finger has to be forced through a narrower space and elicits a snap noise. It is treated with steroid injections.

'Mallet finger'

'Mallet finger' is also called 'baseball finger' (see Fig. 10.15). The extensor tendon is damaged at its insertion into the distal phalanx so that the DIP joint cannot be fully extended. It is treated by splinting the finger with the DIP joint fully extended.

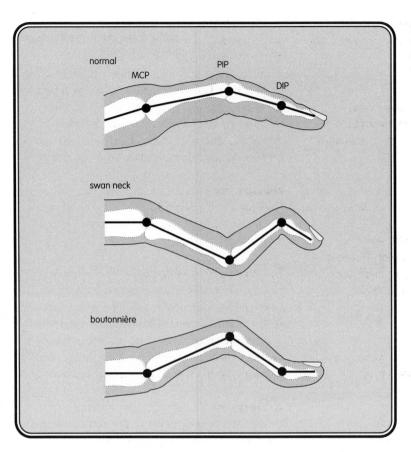

Fig. 10.14 Finger deformities in rheumatoid arthritis: normal finger, swan-neck and boutonnière deformities.

'Dropped finger'

'Dropped finger' is caused by tendon rupture at the wrist—either direct or as a complication of rheumatoid arthritis—resulting in loss of finger extension at the MCP joint.

Ganglia

Aetiology

Ganglia are smooth swellings containing clear viscous fluid which appear as painless lumps on the dorsum of the wrist (Fig. 10.16). They are mostly unilocular, and have walls of fibrous tissue. Ganglia form around the joint capsule and tendon sheath but do not communicate with the joint space.

Management

Ganglia are treated by excision only if they press on the local ulnar or median nerves.

Dupuytren's contracture

Aetiology

In Dupuytren's contracture the palmar aponeurosis is thickened and contracted, and there is skin tethering (Fig. 10.17). Dupuytren's contracture is commonly bilateral, symmetrical, and painless. The fingers become flexed at the MCP and PIP joints. There may be fibrous thickenings in the dorsal knuckle pads (Garod's pads) and on the soles of the feet.

Epidemiology

Dupuytren's contracture affects more men than women, may be familial, and has associations with alcoholism, antiepileptic drugs, and Peyronie's disease (fibrosis of the corpus cavernosum).

Management

Dupuytren's contracture is treated by surgical excision

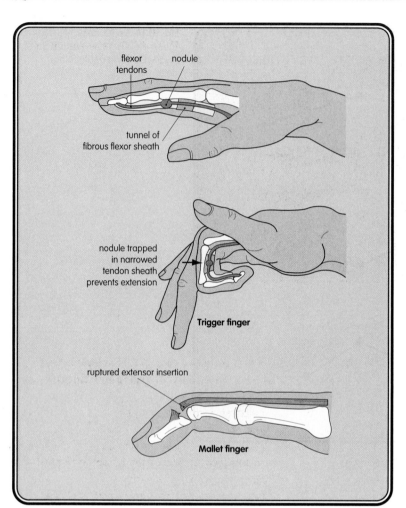

flexor tendons

nodule

tunnel of fibrous flexor sheath

nodule trapped in narrowed tendon sheath prevents extension

Trigger finger

ruptured extensor insertion

Mallet finger

Fig. 10.15 'Trigger finger' and 'mallet finger' due to tendon injuries. See text for details.

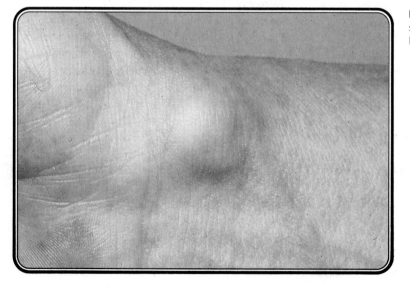

Fig. 10.16 Ganglion at the dorsal surface of the wrist. (Courtesy of Dr J.H. Klippel.)

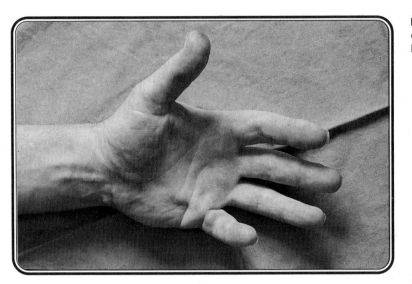

Fig. 10.17 Dupuytren's contracture of the palmar fascia. (Courtesy of Dr J.H. Klippel.)

of the thickened region, only when the deformity is progressive.

Carpal tunnel syndrome

Aetiology
Carpal tunnel syndrome is due to median nerve compression as it passes under the flexor retinaculum. It occurs in premenstrual and pregnant women, and in cases of myxoedema and rheumatoid arthritis.

Clinical features
In carpal tunnel syndrome, there is paraesthesia and pain in the median nerve distribution in the hand (thumb, index, and middle and radial half of the ring finger). Pain is worse at night and after repetitive movements. Later, there is wasting and decreased sensation of the thenar eminence.

Management
Carpal tunnel syndrome is treated either conservatively with diuretics and hydrocortisone injections, or by surgical division of the flexor retinaculum.

Hip joint
Coxa vara
Aetiology
Coxa vara includes any condition in which the angle between the neck and the shaft of the femur is less than the normal 125 degrees (Fig. 10.18). This leads to true shortening of the limb and a limping walk due to a Trendelenburg 'dip'.

The cause of coxa vara may be:
- Congenital.
- A slipped upper femoral epiphysis.
- Fracture (trochanteric with malunion, non-united fractures of the femoral neck).
- Bone-softening (rickets, osteomalacia, or Paget's disease of bone).

Congenital dislocation of the hip
Epidemiology
Congenital dislocation of the hip (CDH) should be diagnosed and corrected in the first week of life to prevent delayed walking and abnormal gait. Girls are eight times more likely to have CDH than boys; the left hip more than the right. The condition occurs more after a breech delivery and if a relative is affected. The acetabulum is abnormally shallow with a very upwardly sloping roof, the femoral head is displaced upwards and laterally, and the joint capsule may fold inwards.

Management
CDH is treated in various ways according to the age of the patient. Treatment may involve splints, joint reduction, osteotomy, or hip displacement.

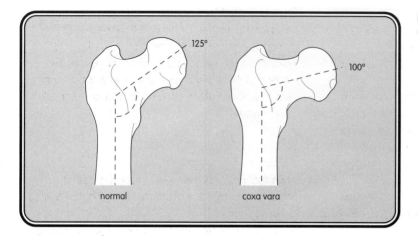

Fig. 10.18 Normal femur and coxa vara.

normal — 125°

coxa vara — 100°

Perthe's disease

Perthe's disease occurs in children and involves osteochondritis of the epiphysis of the femoral head. There is avascular necrosis of unknown cause, resulting in bone fragmentation with concurrent revascularization and new bone formation. There is narrowing of the joint space and flattening of the femoral head, which are risks for early arthritis.

Management

Surgical containment is necessary to treat severe cases of Perthe's disease.

Slipped upper femoral epiphysis

Aetiology

In adolescents, there may be a displacement of the upper epiphysis downward and backward from the femoral neck along the epiphyseal line (Fig. 10.19). This slipped upper femoral epiphysis affects overweight patients and males more than females. There is limping and pain in the groin, thigh, or knee, and limited abduction.

Complications include avascular necrosis and coxa vara.

Management

Slipped upper femoral epiphysis is treated by pinning the femur into position, and osteotomy.

Transient synovitis

Transient synovitis is a short-lived condition of childhood, of unknown aetiology. It causes pain, limping, and limited hip movements. X-rays are normal.

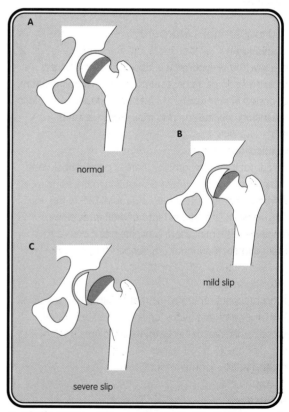

A
normal

B
mild slip

C
severe slip

Fig. 10.19 (A) Normal femoral epiphysis, (B) mild (C) severe slipped upper femoral epiphysis.

Management
No treatment is required for transient synovitis as it recovers spontaneously in about 4 weeks.

Tuberculous arthritis
TB frequently affects the hip joint, causing pain, limping, limited movement, and muscle spasm. X-rays show bone rarefaction (decreased density but normal volume) and subsequent articular cartilage and bony erosion.

Management
Tuberculous arthritis is treated with antituberculous drugs. If the joint has been destroyed, arthrodesis (joint fusion) is performed.

Osteoarthritis of the hip
Aetiology
Osteoarthritis of the hip is a very common cause of disability, especially in the elderly. It may develop from general wear and tear, or as a sequel to acetabular injuries, Perthe's disease, coxa vara, or slipped femoral epiphysis.

Pathology
In osteoarthritis of the hip the articular cartilage is worn away where stress is transmitted. The underlying bone becomes sclerotic and there is cyst formation; there is also synovial hypertrophy, capsular fibrosis, and osteophytes in the joint margins. Pain occurs in the groin and may also radiate to the knee; this is made worse by walking and relieved by rest. All hip movements are limited.

Management
The treatment of osteoarthritis of the hip depends on its severity—either conservatively, i.e. analgesics and hydrocortisone injections, or surgically by osteotomy, joint replacement, or arthrodesis.

Rheumatoid arthritis of the hip
The hip is frequently affected in rheumatoid arthritis. There is progressive femoral head erosion that leads to leg shortening, limited movement, gluteal and thigh muscle wasting, and gradual pain.

Management
Rheumatoid arthritis is treated conservatively with NSAIDs and immunosuppressants or by hip replacement.

Pain referred to the hip
Pain may be referred to the hip from the spine (prolapsed disc, sacro-iliac arthritis), the pelvis and lower abdomen (appendicular abscess, pyosalpinx, irritation of the obturator nerve or muscle spasm), or from thrombosis of the lower abdominal aorta and its main branches.

Gait
Aetiology
Abnormal gait may arise when there is a loss of coordination in the movements of the spine, hip, knee, ankle, and foot.

There are several types of abnormal gait, including:
- Osteogenic gait—bone shortening leads to limping.
- Arthrogenic gait—ankylosis; fixed flexion deformity making one or both buttocks prominent, and abduction deformity where a leg swings round during walking.
- Myogenic gait—weak gluteal muscles in muscular dystrophy giving a waddling gait.
- Neurogenic gait—disorders such as hemiparesis, cerebellar ataxia, parkinsonism, cerebral palsy, footdrop, and bilateral leg spasticity all show characteristic gaits.

Knee
Genu varum and genu valgum
Aetiology and epidemiology
Genu varum (bow legs) and genu valgum (knock knees) commonly occur in childhood, and usually correct spontaneously (Fig. 10.20). They may also occur secondary to injury or disease (fractures, rheumatoid arthritis or osteoarthritis, rickets, osteomalacia, Paget's disease of bone).

Meniscal tears
Epidemiology
Meniscal tears are common in young men. They are usually caused by a twisting injury, especially in sport.

Aetiology
The medial meniscus is torn more often than the lateral. When the meniscus splits longitudinally a 'bucket-handle' tear occurs, where the meniscus remains attached at both ends; if either end becomes detached, 'anterior horn' or 'posterior horn' tears are produced (Fig. 10.21). The torn tags may either cause mechanical 'locking' of the

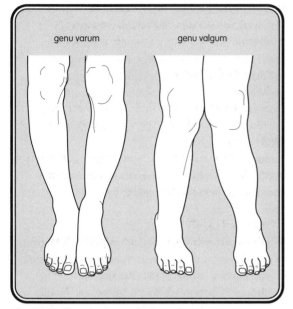

genu varum   genu valgum

Fig. 10.20 Genu varum and genu valgum.

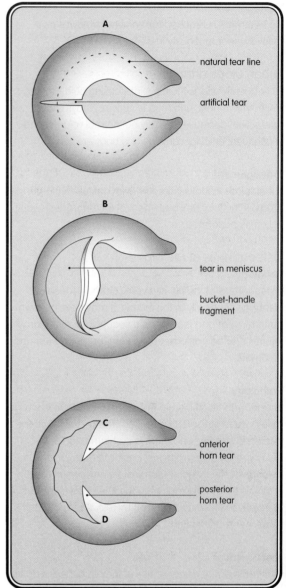

A

natural tear line

artificial tear

B

tear in meniscus

bucket-handle
fragment

C

anterior
horn tear

posterior
horn tear

D

Fig. 10.21 Pattern of meniscal tears: (A) the natural tear line,
(B) 'bucket-handle tear' (the most common type), anterior
horn tear (C) and posterior horn tear (D).

knee by becoming jammed between the tibia and femur
(preventing full extension) or predispose to secondary
osteoarthritis because of the irritation to the joint.

Management
Meniscal tears are treated by arthroscopic excision of
the displaced tag.

Meniscal cysts
Aetiology
Meniscal cysts are similar to ganglia and develop from
the lateral joint line. They may either arise from a
previous joint injury or occur spontaneously. The
swelling is usually most painful at night.

Management
Meniscal cysts are treated by excision.

Osteochondritis dissecans
Aetiology
Osteochondritis dissecans is local ischaemic necrosis
of bone and articular cartilage. It affects the knee more
than any other joint. Osteochondral fragmentation
produces loose bodies in the joint capsule.

Other causes of loose bodies in the knee include
osteoarthritis, fracture of the joint surface, and synovial
chondromatosis.

Recurrent dislocation of the patella
Aetiology
The patella is always displaced laterally when the

knee is flexed. Predisposing factors for recurrent dislocation of the patella include generalized ligament laxity, anatomical abnormalities of the patella or lateral condyle of the femur, or a genu valgum deformity. Recurrent dislocation of the patella tends to affect adolescent girls, often bilaterally.

Clinical features

In recurrent dislocation of the patella there is severe pain in the front of the knee so that the patient cannot extend the joint and may collapse. Repeated dislocations can predispose to the development of osteoarthritis.

Management

Recurrent dislocation of the patella is treated by strengthening the quadriceps muscle (especially vastus medialis muscle). If this fails, the joint needs to be stabilized surgically.

Chondromalacia patellae
Aetiology

Softening of the patellar articular cartilage, or chondromalacia patellae, is an important cause of anterior knee pain, especially in teenage girls. Pain is worse on climbing up and down stairs, and there may be joint effusion.

Management

Chondromalacia patellae is treated with analgesics and by strengthening the vastus medialis muscle; surgical correction is often unsuccessful.

Osteoarthritis of the knee
Aetiology

The knee is affected by osteoarthritis more than other joints, especially in overweight patients with a long-standing genu varum deformity.

Clinical features

Characteristic features of osteoarthritis of the knee include articular cartilage breakdown, subchondral bone sclerosis, and peripheral osteophyte formation. There is joint pain on use, and swelling, leading to knee locking. The quadriceps muscle is usually wasted.

Management

Treatment of osteoarthritis of the knee depends on the

severity of the disease. It may be treated conservatively with analgesics and physiotherapy, or surgically by débridement, osteotomy, or joint replacement.

Bursitis of the knee
Pathology

Bursae can become inflamed because of infection, trauma, or repeated irritating friction giving rise to swelling and effusion.

The prepatellar bursa ('housemaid's knee'), infrapatellar bursa ('vicar's knee'), and semimembranosus bursa (popliteal cyst) are commonly affected.

Ankle and foot
Congenital club foot (talipes equinovarus)
Pathology

Congenital club foot shows as foot inversion, medial inversion (adduction), and plantarflexion (Fig. 10.22). The calf and peroneal muscles are also underdeveloped.

Boys are affected by congenital club foot more than girls. The condition may be associated with spina bifida.

Management

Congenital club foot is corrected by splinting and/or surgery.

Pes planus and pes cavus

Pes planus (flat foot) is a flattened longitudinal arch causing the medial border of the foot almost to touch the ground (Fig. 10.23). It can be caused by underlying general joint laxity. Often there are no symptoms, but there may be foot strain and osteoarthritis of the tarsal joints in later life.

Pes cavus (hollow foot) is a high longitudinal arch, which may be congenital or associated with neurological disorders, leading to weak intrinsic muscles (see Fig. 10.23). The toes may be clawed and the metatarsal heads prominent as they are weightbearing.

Hammer toes
Clinical features

In hammer toes, the toes are flexed at the PIP joint and extended at the MTP joint (Fig. 10.24). The second toes are most commonly affected.

Management

Hammer toes are treated by lengthening the tendons and excising the MTP joint (see Fig. 10.24).

159

Claw toes

Clinical features

In claw toes, the toes are flexed at both the PIP and DIP joints, and extended at the MTP joint (see Fig. 10.24). Claw toes occur in rheumatoid arthritis and after poliomyelitis.

Management

Claw toes are treated by a flexor–extensor transfer operation.

Mallet toes

Clinical features

In mallet toes, there is damage to the extensor tendon at its insertion into the distal phalanx. The DIP joint cannot be extended fully.

Management

Mallet toes are treated by placing a splint onto the toe, with the DIP joint fully extended.

Hallux valgus

In hallus valgus, the big toe deviates laterally at the MTP joint, which develops a protective bursa (bunion) where the shoe rubs. This condition may lead to hammer toes, bursitis, metatarsalgia, and secondary osteoarthritis of the MTP joint.

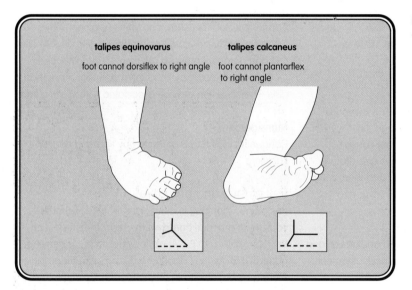

Fig. 10.22 Features of talipes equinovarus and talipes calcaneus.

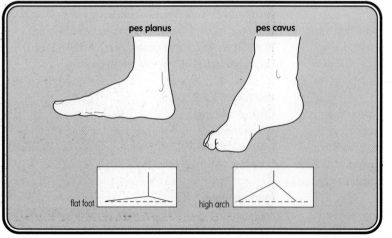

Fig. 10.23 Features of pes planus and pes cavus.

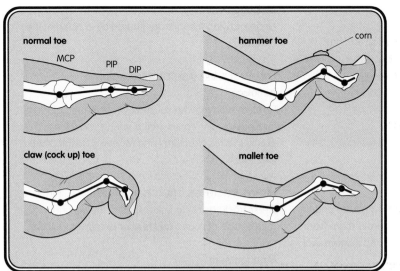

Fig. 10.24 Toe deformitites: normal toe, 'claw toe', and 'mallet toe'.

normal toe

MCP

PIP DIP

hammer toe

corn

claw (cock up) toe

mallet toe

The wearing of high heels with pointed toes may contribute to this deformity; it is seen in elderly women.

Hallux rigidus
Aetiology
Joint stiffness in the big toe, or hallus rigidus, may be due to osteoarthritis of the MTP joint, trauma, osteochondritis dissecans in the head of the first metatarsal bone, or gout. There is pain on walking and limited movement.

Epidemiology
Men are more commonly affected with hallus rigidus than women.

Management
Treatment of hallus rigidus involves dealing with the underlying cause, then replacing the joint if necessary.

Toenail lesions
Ingrown toenails
Aetiology
Ingrown toenails are nails that have become embedded in the lateral skin folds and formed inflamed (sometimes pus-filled) ulcerations.

Ingrown toenails can be prevented by the correct cutting of the nails.

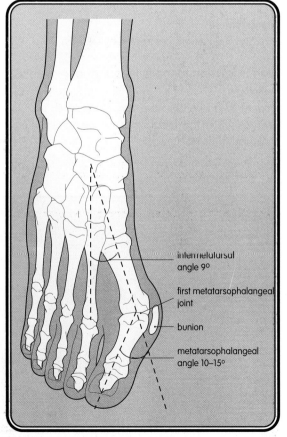

intermetatarsal angle 9°

first metatarsophalangeal joint

bunion

metatarsophalangeal angle 10–15°

Fig. 10.25 Hallux valgus.

A Baker's cyst is a herniation of the joint synovium backwards and downwards; it is not the same as a popliteal cyst.

Management
Ingrown toenails are treated by inserting gauze under the ingrowing edges of the nail to separate them from the skin fold, or by removal of the nail and its germinal matrix.

Overgrowing toenails (onychogryphosis)
Aetiology
Overgrowing toenails are very thick, hard, and curved laterally (Fig. 10.26).

Management
Overgrowing toenails are treated by excision.

Undergrowing toenails (subungual exostosis)
Aetiology
Undergrowing toenails have a bony outgrowth (exostosis) from the dorsal surface of the distal phalanx, that pushes the nail upwards.

Management
Undergrowing toenails are treated by excision of the exostosis.

Forefoot pain (metatarsalgia)
Aetiology
Forefoot pain may be caused by foot or toe deformities (pes planus, pes cavus, hallux valgus, claw toes); it also occurs in stress fractures and Morton's metatarsalgia (Fig. 10.27).

Stress fractures (march fractures)
Stress fractures occur in the shaft of the second or third metatarsals of young adults after excessive walking.

Management
Stress fractures are treated by rest and wearing a plaster during healing.

Morton's metatarsalgia (plantar digital neuritis)
Morton's metatarsalgia is the presence of a fibrous thickening of a digital nerve between the metatarsals. Wearing shoes causes compressional pain in this region, which then radiates to the third and fourth toes.

Management
Morton's metatarsalgia is treated by wearing rubber pads in shoes or excising the thickened nerve segment.

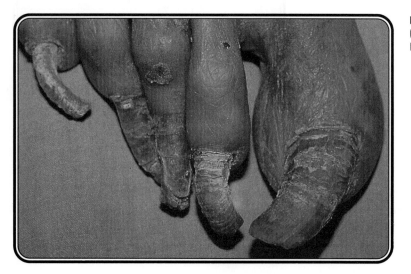

Fig. 10.26 Overgrown toenails. (Courtesy of Dr G. White, and the Department of Dermatology, UCSD.)

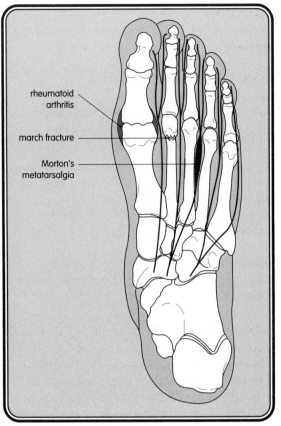

rheumatoid
arthritis

march fracture

Morton's
metatarsalgia

Fig. 10.27 Causes of forefoot pain.

Rheumatoid arthritis in the ankle and foot

Rheumatoid arthritis affects the ankle and foot joints in a similar way to the wrist and hands, with the added complication that the patient must walk on them.

There is subluxation of the metatarsal heads, with hallux valgus, clawed toes, and prominent calluses causing pain.

Name some of the conditions (describing the aetiology and management) involving:

- **Disorders of the back.**
- **Disorders of the shoulder and elbow joint.**
- **Disorders of the hip joint.**
- **Disorders of the knee, ankle, and foot.**

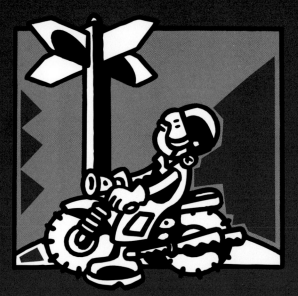

SELF-ASSESSMENT

Multiple-choice Questions

Indicate whether each answer is true or false.

1. In an action potential:

(a) Size is proportional to the stimulus strength.
(b) Initiation occurs when the membrane potential is reduced to a critical value.
(c) Influx of sodium ions is responsible for the rising phase.
(d) There is a transient decrease in membrane permeability of potassium ions.
(e) The duration and size are constant for all cell types.

2. Recognized side effects of local anaesthetics include:

(a) Allergic reactions causing sudden collapse.
(b) Stimulation of the central nervous system.
(c) Constriction of blood vessels.
(d) Physical dependency.
(e) Hypertension.

3. Neurotransmission at the neuromuscular junction is impaired by:

(a) Hemicholinium.
(b) Suxamethonium.
(c) Adrenaline.
(d) Botulinum toxin.
(e) Edrophonium.

4. Edrophonium:

(a) Is used in the treatment of myasthenia gravis.
(b) May cause constriction of the pupil.
(c) Is an anticholinesterase.
(d) Impairs neuromuscular transmission.
(e) Decreases acetylcholine release at the neuromuscular junction.

5. The RMP of a nerve fibre:

(a) Has a higher concentration of potassium ions inside the nerve than on the outside.
(b) When reduced, results in an increase in excitability of the cell.
(c) Has a value of –90 mV in muscle cells.
(d) Is also known as the equilibrium potential.
(e) Is equal to the equilibrium potential of potassium.

6. Cartilage:

(a) Is an avascular tissue.
(b) Never forms permanent structures.
(c) Can increase in size by appositional and interstitial growth.
(d) Can survive if invaded by ingrowing capillaries.
(e) Is always covered by perichondrium.

7. Smooth muscle cells:

(a) Have a single nucleus located at the widest part of the cell.
(b) Contain myofilaments thath can only be seen with an electron microscope.
(c) Cannot be replaced in adult life by the transformation of mesenchymal cells.
(d) Remain a constant size throughout life.
(e) Form tight junctions with each other.

8. Hyaline cartilage:

(a) Contains prominent elastic fibres.
(b) Contains a few collagen-like fibres.
(c) Is the precursor of endochondral ossification.
(d) Forms the knee menisci.
(e) Is vascular compared with bone.

9. Long bones:

(a) Usually ossify directly from mesenchyme.
(b) Are made wholly of compact bone.
(c) Normally contain yellow marrow in adulthood.
(d) Are organized in haversian systems.
(e) Are covered with an acellular periosteum.

10. Endochondral ossification:

(a) Occurs in all long bones except the clavicle.
(b) Occurs in cartilage that has replaced a membranous model.
(c) Has its primary centres appearing *in utero*.
(d) Is usually complete by the age of 25 years.
(e) Is typical in the bones of the skull.

11. In the development of long bones:

(a) Osteoclasts do not absorb the calcified matrix of the cartilage.
(b) Osteoblasts become osteocytes.
(c) Endochondral ossification extends along the diaphysis.
(d) The epiphyseal plate separates the diaphysis from the metaphysis.
(e) Circumferential growth is by subperiosteal ossification.

12. The epiphyses:

(a) Are all present at birth.
(b) Are formed in hyaline cartilage.
(c) Are not present in all long bones.
(d) Are involved in increasing length and width of long bones.
(e) May occur at sites of muscle attachment.

13. In synovial joints:

(a) Articular surfaces are always lined by articular cartilage.
(b) Fibrocartilaginous discs usually partially divide the joint cavity.
(c) The hinged type can be exemplified by metacarpophalangeal joints.
(d) The stability of the joint is generally inversely proportional to its mobility.
(e) The hip joint is of the plane type.

14. Striated muscle:

(a) Contains alternating A and Z bands.
(b) Fibres are multinucleate.
(c) Is present in the upper part of the oesophagus.
(d) Fibres are bound together by sarcolemma.
(e) Is the most common type of muscle found in the body.

15. Collagen:

(a) Is formed by undifferentiated mesenchymal cells.
(b) Is normally embedded in ground substance.
(c) Has a breakdown product called hydroxyproline, excreted in the urine.
(d) Type III is found in the basement membrane of most cells.
(e) Fibres are mostly located intracellularly.

16. The destruction of bone is associated with the following biochemical changes:

(a) Raised urinary hydroxyproline.
(b) Raised plasma alkaline phosphatase.
(c) Raised plasma acid phosphatase.
(d) Raised plasma calcium.
(e) Lowered plasma phosphate.

17. Osteoporosis differs from osteomalacia in the following ways:

(a) The density of the skeleton is reduced in osteoporosis and not in osteomalacia.
(b) The remaining bone in osteoporosis has a normal histological appearance.
(c) There are gross changes in the epiphyses in osteomalacia.
(d) Pseudofractures are more common in osteoporosis than in osteomalacia.
(e) Excess bone matrix is found in osteomalacia.

18. The following promote fracture healing:

(a) Absence of infection.
(b) Adequate vitamin C.
(c) Good blood supply.
(d) Immediate mobilization.
(e) Treatment with steroids.

19. Metastases in bone show the following characteristic features:

(a) Both bone destruction and new bone formation.
(b) Pathological fractures.
(c) Lowered plasma alkaline phosphatase.
(d) Red marrow affected more than yellow marrow.
(e) Red blood cells in peripheral blood may be of immature forms.

20. Calcium:

(a) Controls neuromuscular excitability.
(b) Acts as an intracellular second messenger.
(c) Is mobilized slowly from cancellous bone to blood.
(d) Absorption in small intestine is enhanced by vitamin D.
(e) Excess in blood is reduced by parathyroid hormone.

21. The following properties hold true for all three types of muscle:

(a) Rapid stimulation results in summation.
(b) An increase in intracellular calcium concentration is necessary for muscular contraction.
(c) Contraction is controlled by the nervous system.
(d) Membrane depolarization is necessary for APs to occur.
(e) The presence of actin and myosin.

22. The following statements are correct:

(a) Intercalated discs are present in skeletal muscle.
(b) Cardiac muscle fibres are cross-striated.
(c) Transverse tubules are found in smooth muscle.
(d) Myofilaments are arranged in an organized way in smooth muscle.
(e) Muscle spindles are present in smooth muscle.

23. In cardiac muscle:

(a) The AP is initiated in the sino-atrial node.
(b) The AP is shorter than that in skeletal muscle.
(c) The AP demonstrates a plateau phase.
(d) Cells are multinucleated.
(e) Summation of contractions does not occur.

24. Regarding the AP in ventricular cardiac muscle:

(a) Calcium ions are responsible for the rising phase of the AP.
(b) The refractory period is longer than that following an AP in skeletal muscle.
(c) The sympathetic nervous system shortens the plateau phase of the AP.
(d) Calcium ions play a part in the AP.
(e) Initiation is neurogenic.

25. In smooth muscle cells:

(a) The protein desmin is present.
(b) The protein troponin is present.
(c) Sodium ions are responsible for the AP.
(d) Contraction requires lower ATP contraction.
(e) The protein calmodulin is a component of the thin filament.

26. In skeletal muscle contraction, ATP:

(a) Is required to cause detachment of myosin heads from the actin filaments.
(b) Is provided by glycolysis.
(c) Is produced by slow synthesis from creatine kinase.
(d) Is necessary for the influx of sodium ions.
(e) Is produced by oxidative phosphorylation.

27. Upon contraction of skeletal muscle:

(a) The rise in intracellular calcium ions results from direct entry through the cell membrane.
(b) The calcium ions bind to tropomyosin.
(c) The number of sarcomeres decreases.
(d) The actin and myosin filaments shorten.
(e) The strength of contraction is influenced by initial muscle fibre length.

28. With regard to the arrangement of skeletal muscles:

(a) Muscles are arranged in groups.
(b) A muscle may be a member of only one group.
(c) For a given volume of muscle, an oblique arrangement of muscle fibres would result in a greater force of contraction than a parallel arrangement.
(d) Muscle fibres are innervated by muscle spindles.
(e) The origin of a muscle is the attachment site at which there is little movement when the muscle performs its main action.

29. With regard to saltatory conduction:

(a) It can occur in unmyelinated nerve fibres.
(b) Speed is proportional to the diameter of the nerve fibre.
(c) Speed is proportional to the strength of local circuits.
(d) A large safety factor is demonstrated.
(e) Membrane depolarization does not occur.

30. With regard to skeletal muscle:

(a) A smaller stimulus is required to cause local contraction it applied to the Z band.
(b) Distance between the Z bands is constant during contraction.
(c) Each muscle fibre is innervated by only one motor neuron.
(d) APs are propagated in both directions to the ends of the muscle fibre.
(e) The length of the I bands decreases during contraction.

31. With regard to the motor unit:

(a) The muscle fibres within a motor unit lie side by side.
(b) The muscle fibres within a motor unit are of the same type.
(c) Muscles involved in fine movement have smaller motor units.
(d) The strength of muscle contraction is increased by recruiting more motor units.
(e) The muscle fibres within a motor unit contract simultaneously.

32. HLA B27 may be associated with the following:

(a) Rheumatoid arthritis.
(b) Osteoarthritis.
(c) Reiter's syndrome.
(d) Behçet's syndrome.
(e) Ankylosing spondylitis.

33. Rheumatoid arthritis:

(a) Is more common in males.
(b) May be complicated by septic arthritis.
(c) Most commonly affects the distal interphalangeal joints.
(d) Is associated with destruction of cartilage.
(e) Patients may demonstrate the presence of ANAs.

34. Myasthenia gravis:

(a) May be associated with ptosis.
(b) Occurs most commonly in the fifth decade.
(c) Is associated with antibodies to ACh.
(d) Is inherited in an autosomal recessive manner.
(e) May be transient in newborn babies of female sufferers.

35. The following statements are correct:

(a) Gower's sign is a feature of myotonic dystrophy.
(b) Duchenne muscular dystrophy is inherited in an autosomal recessive manner.
(c) Fascioscapulohumeral dystrophy may be associated with winging of the scapulae.
(d) Mitochondrial myopathy may be associated with patients infected with HIV.
(e) Pseudohypertrophy of the calves is a sign of Duchenne muscular dystrophy.

36. With regard to muscle function:

(a) Isometric contraction of skeletal muscle is contraction at a constant tension.
(b) The treppe effect is associated with cardiac contraction.
(c) The force of skeletal muscle contraction increases with frequency of stimulation.
(d) Plasticity may involve altering vascular supply to the muscle.
(e) Most muscles in the body are at optimum length for maximal tension.

37. Conduction velocity:

(a) Increases in the presence of a myelin sheath.
(b) Increases up to a temperature of 60°.
(c) Decreases with larger fibre diameters.
(d) Is influenced by the strength of local circuits.
(e) May be less than 1 m/s.

38. Chemical synapses differ from electrical in that:

(a) Transmission is more rapid.
(b) Synaptic cleft is larger.
(c) Plasticity may occur.
(d) They are more common in the body.
(e) Amplification of the signal is possible.

39. The following proteins are components of the thin filament:

(a) Actin.
(b) Desmin.
(c) Calmodulin.
(d) Troponin.
(e) α-Actinin.

40. With regard to muscle fibre types:

(a) Speed of contraction is greatest with red fibres.
(b) Red fibres are resistant to fatigue.
(c) Myoglobin is present in red fibres.
(d) White fibres are involved in maintenance of posture.
(e) Glycogen content is high in white fibres.

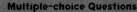

41. In connective tissue:

(a) Ground substance is not part of the extracellular matrix.
(b) There is a low matrix:cell ratio.
(c) There may be undifferentiated mesenchymal cells present.
(d) Elastic fibres are arranged in random sheets.
(e) Proteoglycans are protein chains bound to branched polysaccharides.

42. The skeleton:

(a) Is derived from the primitive mesenchyme.
(b) Has a solid extracellular matrix.
(c) Consists of bone only.
(d) Is a major storage site for calcium.
(e) Does not contain any red bone marrow in adults.

43. Fibrous joints:

(a) Contain fibrous tissue on their articulating surfaces.
(b) Have a joint cavity.
(c) Allow little or no movement.
(d) Of the suture type may become ossified.
(e) Of the syndesmosis type are found in the interosseous membrane of the radioulnar joint.

44. Cartilaginous joints:

(a) Contain some hyaline cartilage.
(b) Of the primary type are all temporary unions.
(c) Of the secondary type are also united by fibrocartilage.
(d) Are generally very mobile.
(e) Are found in the symphysis pubis, costosternal, and manubriosternal joints.

45. A joint:

(a) Allows mobility in direct proportion to its stability.
(b) Has a poor blood supply inside its capsule.
(c) Contains veins and lymphatic vessels in the synovial membrane.
(d) Is supplied by the same nerves as those of the overlying skin and muscles moving the joint.
(e) Does not mediate pain but allows proprioception only.

46. Synovial joints:

(a) Do not always contain a cavity.
(b) Are the most common joint type found in the skeleton.
(c) Of the hinge type allow biaxial movement.
(d) Of the condyloid type are found at the base of the fingers and toes.
(e) Of the ball and socket type allow the greatest range of movement.

47. The human skeleton:

(a) Is bilaterally symmetrical.
(b) Has an axial part, comprising the bones of the head, neck, and trunk.
(c) Has an appendicular part consisting of limb bones only.
(d) Contains active red bone marrow in both children and adults.
(e) Contains bones that all start as a cartilage template.

48. In motor control:

(a) The three main central controls are the cerebral cortex, brainstem, and spinal cord.
(b) The cerebellum and basal ganglia are independent of the cerebral cortex in coordinating movement.
(c) The pyramidal tracts mostly stay on the same side from the motor cortex down the spinal cord.
(d) Muscle spindles are modified muscle fibres called extrafusal fibres.
(e) Golgi tendon organs lie in series with extrafusal muscle fibres.

49. Cartilage:

(a) Consists of chondroblasts and chondrocytes embedded in a cartilage matrix.
(b) Growth and maturation is mainly towards the periphery of the cartilage mass.
(c) Contains a rich blood supply.
(d) Of the hyaline type is present in the epiphyseal plates.
(e) Of the elastic type is found in the epiglottis.

50. Long bones:

(a) Have a shaft called the diaphysis.
(b) Have two expanded ends called metaphyses.
(c) Contain a central medullary cavity.
(d) Consist of compact bone only.
(e) Are lined by endostium.

1. List the location and the function of the five main types of collagen.

2. Write briefly on the functions of the skeleton.

3. Draw the AP produced in nerve fibres. Explain the ions involved at each stage.

4. Briefly describe the differences in the ionic composition of the intra- and extracellular fluid of muscle cells.

5. Write brief notes on fracture healing and how it may be delayed.

6. Draw a sarcomere:
   (a) In relaxed muscle.
   (b) During contraction.

7. Write briefly on the initiation of contraction in smooth muscle.

8. Draw a normal synovial joint.

9. List the extra-articular features of rheumatoid arthritis.

10. List five clinical features of rickets.

11. Draw the sino-atrial node action potential and briefly mention the ions responsible for each phase.

12. What are the five changes that may occur in bone secondary to osteoarthritis?

13. What are the three stages by which muscle fibres are replaced in the adult with an intact basal lamina following damage?

14. Describe three differences between the AP in skeletal muscle and that in the nerve.

15. Describe five differences between slow, fast non-fatiguable, and fast fatiguable motor units.

16. Draw a muscle spindle to show the types of intrafusal fibres.

17. Draw a diagram of a long bone and label the important features.

18. List the blood supply, lymphatic drainage, and nerve supply of bone.

19. Write short notes on periosteum and endosteum.

20. List the differences in histology and location of hyaline and elastic cartilage.

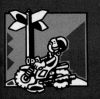

Essay Questions

1. List the events occurring at the NMJ on arrival of an AP at the nerve terminal, and discuss the drugs that may influence this process.

2. Describe the ionic basis of the RMP and how this is maintained.

3. Compare the cardiac AP with that seen in skeletal muscle and explain how any differences may be related to function.

4. Discuss the role of vitamin D, PTH, and calcitonin in calcium metabolism.

5. Compare and contrast intramembranous ossification with endochondral ossification.

6. Describe the microstructure of skeletal muscle.

7. Describe the epidemiology, pathology, and clinical features of osteoporosis.

8. What are the clinical manifestations of osteoarthritis in the wrist and hand? Compare these with the 'rheumatoid hand'.

9. Write an essay on the microscopic arrangement of bone.

10. Describe the epidemiology, pathology, and clinical features of Duchenne muscular dystrophy.

MCQ Answers

1. (a)F, (b)T, (c)T, (d)T, (e)F
2. (a)T, (b)T, (c)F, (d)F, (e)F
3. (a)T, (b)T, (c)F, (d)T, (e)F
4. (a)T, (b)T, (c)T, (d)F, (e)F
5. (a)T, (b)T, (c)T, (d)T, (e)T
6. (a)T, (b)F, (c)T, (d)F, (e)F
7. (a)T, (b)T, (c)F, (d)F, (e)T
8. (a)F, (b)T, (c)T, (d)F, (e)F
9. (a)F, (b)F, (c)T, (d)T, (e)F
10. (a)T, (b)T, (c)T, (d)T, (e)F
11. (a)F, (b)T, (c)T, (d)F, (e)T
12. (a)F, (b)T, (c)F, (d)F, (e)T
13. (a)F, (b)F, (c)F, (d)T, (e)F
14. (a)F, (b)T, (c)T, (d)F, (e)T
15. (a)F, (b)T, (c)T, (d)F, (e)F
16. (a)T, (b)T, (c)F, (d)T, (e)T
17. (a)F, (b)T, (c)T, (d)F, (e)T
18. (a)T, (b)T, (c)T, (d)F, (e)F
19. (a)T, (b)T, (c)F, (d)T, (e)T
20. (a)T, (b)T, (c)F, (d)T, (e)F
21. (a)F, (b)T, (c)F, (d)T, (e)T
22. (a)F, (b)T, (c)F, (d)F, (e)F
23. (a)T, (b)F, (c)T, (d)F, (e)T
24. (a)F, (b)T, (c)T, (d)T, (e)F
25. (a)T, (b)F, (c)F, (d)T, (e)F

26. (a)T, (b)T, (c)F, (d)T, (e)T
27. (a)F, (b)F, (c)F, (d)F, (e)T
28. (a)T, (b)F, (c)T, (d)F, (e)T
29. (a)F, (b)T, (c)T, (d)T, (e)F
30. (a)T, (b)T, (c)T, (d)T, (e)T
31. (a)F, (b)T, (c)T, (d)T, (e)T
32. (a)F, (b)F, (c)T, (d)F, (e)T
33. (a)F, (b)T, (c)F, (d)T, (e)T
34. (a)T, (b)F, (c)F, (d)F, (e)T
35. (a)F, (b)F, (c)T, (d)T, (e)T
36. (a)F, (b)T, (c)T, (d)T, (e)T
37. (a)T, (b)F, (c)F, (d)T, (e)T
38. (a)F, (b)T, (c)T, (d)T, (e)T
39. (a)T, (b)F, (c)F, (d)T, (e)T
40. (a)F, (b)T, (c)T, (d)F, (e)T
41. (a)F, (b)F, (c)T, (d)T, (e)T
42. (a)T, (b)T, (c)F, (d)T, (e)F
43. (a)T, (b)F, (c)T, (d)T, (e)T
44. (a)T, (b)F, (c)T, (d)F, (e)T
45. (a)F, (b)F, (c)T, (d)T, (e)F
46. (a)F, (b)T, (c)F, (d)T, (e)T
47. (a)T, (b)T, (c)F, (d)T, (e)F
48. (a)T, (b)F, (c)F, (d)F, (e)T
49. (a)T, (b)F, (c)F, (d)T, (e)T
50. (a)T, (b)F, (c)T, (d)F, (e)T

1. Refer to Fig. 1.4.

2. The skeleton performs several functions. These include:
   - Support.
   - Protection of organs.
   - Mechanical basis for locomotion.
   - Storage of minerals.
   - Haematopoiesis.

3. Refer to Fig. 2.13.

4. Refer to Fig. 2.11. The cell membrane is selectively permeable to K^+ and Cl^- and the presence of intracellular impermeant ions; it is relatively impermeable to Na^+.

5. Fracture healing involves several stages. These include:
   - A haematoma forming at the fracture site, which then forms into a procallus; this procallus is converted into a fibrocartilaginous callus.
   - The fibrocartilaginous callus forming an osseous callus (trabecular lamellar bone); remodelling takes place by osteoclasts.
   - Delay; this can be caused by several factors such as malalignment, movement during healing, poor blood supply, and soft tissue interposition in the fracture gap.

6. Refer to Fig. 2.8.

7. The initiation of contraction in smooth muscle takes place in three ways. These are:
   - Autonomic nervous system stimulation. You need to mention varicosities, release of neurotransmitter, and the fact that receptor activatation may result in excitation or inhibition. Examples of neurotransmitters are ACh or noradrenaline.
   - Circulating hormones. Examples of circulating hormones include ACh, adrenaline, noradrenaline, angiotensin, vasopressin, serotonin, and histamine. These hormones act by direct opening/closing of ion channels and activation of second messenger systems. Hormones are excitatory or inhibitory.
   - Local tissue factors. Refer to Fig. 2.43. The mechanism for this is unknown.

8. Refer to Fig. 3.18

9. Refer to Fig. 10.3.

10. The five clinical features of rickets include:
    - Bowing of the legs.
    - Rachitic rosary, i.e. an overgrowth of costochondral junctions.
    - Flattened, bossed, square skull.
    - Expansion of the metaphyses, producing large wrists.
    - Proximal myopathy.

    Other features include short stature, delayed closure of the anterior fontanelle, and delayed dentition.

11. Refer to Fig. 2.36.

12. The five changes that may occur in bone secondary to osteoarthritis include:
    - Eburnation, i.e. thickening and polishing of subarticular bone due to bone–bone articulation.
    - Disuse muscle atrophy due to immobility of a joint.
    - Synovial hyperplasia resulting from inflammation.
    - Subchondral cyst formation.
    - Formation of osteophytes.

13. There are three stages by which muscle fibres are replaced in the adult with an intact basal lamina following damage, namely:
    - Satellite cells (small spindle-shaped cells located between sarcolemma and basal lamina) proliferate to form myoblasts.
    - Myotubes are formed by fusion of myoblasts.
    - Resulting new muscle fibres have abnormally placed central nuclei.

14. The three differences between the AP in skeletal muscle and that in the nerve are:
    - Conduction velocity. In skeletal muscle this is 3–5 m/s while in nerve it is variable (from <1 to 100 m/s).
    - Duration. In skeletal muscle this is 1–5 ms while in nerve it is < 1 ms.
    - RMP. In skeletal muscle this is –80 to –90 mV while in nerve it is –40 mV (in small-diameter nerves) to –90 mV (in large-diameter nerves).

    In addition, the presence of T tubules in skeletal muscle enables the spread of an AP to the cell interior, whereas in nerves, membrane depolarization is sufficient.

15. Refer to Fig. 2.25.
    Highlight the fibre diameter, force of contraction, function, capillaries, and source of energy.

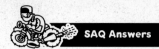

16. Refer to Fig. 4.3.

17. Refer to Fig. 3.4

18. Periosteal arteries supply blood to compact bone, nutrient arteries to spongy bone and bone marrow, metaphyseal arteries to the metaphysis, and epiphyseal arteries to the epiphysis. Veins accompany these arteries.

The lymph drainage of bone occurs mainly from the periosteum towards the regional lymph nodes.

Vasomotor nerves accompany blood vessels to bone, while periosteal nerves carry pain fibres.

19. Periosteum lines the outer surface of bone. It comprises two layers—the outer layer contains blood vessels, nerves, and lymphatics and the inner layer contains osteoblasts and osteoclasts.

Endosteum lines the inner surface of bone. It comprises a single layer that contains osteoblasts and osteoclasts.

20. Hyaline cartilage is composed predominantly of type II collagen regularly arranged along lines of stress; it has an amorphous matrix. Hyaline cartilage is found in the epiglottis, external auditory meatus, auditory tube, and auricle of the ear.

Elastic cartilage is mainly composed of elastic fibres and elastic lamellae; it has very little matrix. Elastic cartilage is found in discs of temporomandibular and sternoclavicular joints and also on the articular surface of the clavicle and mandible.

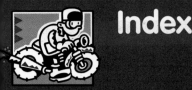

Index

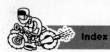

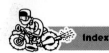

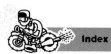

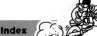

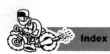

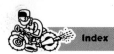

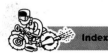

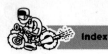